Free to Speak II
Successful Long Term Management
of Spasmodic Dysphonia

D0782908

ISBN: 1-4392-7267-0
ISBN-13: 9781439272671

Free to Speak II
Successful Long Term Management
of Spasmodic Dysphonia

Holistic Voice Rehabilitation

Connie M. Pike, M.A., CCC-SLP

2010

Dedication and Acknowledgements

This book is dedicated to the memory of my son, Taylor Keith Pike, born November 9, 1985. Taylor's spirit left his earthly body to soar into the heavens on May 14, 2007. It was an adventure to be Taylor's mom for 21 years. I miss him every day.

I would also like to acknowledge my husband, Bob, who "covered" for me with love and patience when I had no voice and who always knows the right words to say to my patients. His presence at the clinics is a wonderful support.

I am grateful for my daughter, Megan, who graces us with her beautiful smile and kind words whenever she can. I appreciate her support and comments on the book project and her encouragement that I keep moving forward even in the face of critics. Bob, Taylor, and Megan always believed I could make a difference in the world.

I am eternally grateful for the Spirit of God, which lives in me, and gives me mercy and grace each and every day if I only turn my heart to Him. My strength and wisdom come only through the gifts He has given me.

I also want to acknowledge my long-time friend, Nancy Helms Woods, who took on the job of creative editor and to Dr. Ronald W. Cox, associate professor at Florida International University, for completing several preliminary reviews of the text and for his valuable comments.

Finally, I owe a debt of gratitude for every person with Spasmodic Dysphonia who took a chance on me and came to me for help. I have learned from each of you and you are the new pioneers in the SD world. Go and conquer this dreadful condition and be a beacon of light for the next generation.

Contents

FREE TO SPEAK II: SUCCESSFUL LONG-TERM MANAGEMENT OF SPASMODIC DYSPHONIA
Preface

The phone rings. I glance at the caller ID. Unknown caller or out of area calls are ignored by choice, not necessity. I answer other calls with ease and confidence, knowing I can handle any matter at hand without choking or being asked if I am sick or to repeat myself.

My computer is on the blink. I call customer support and plead my case for resolution. It takes more than an hour. It is annoying, and perhaps there is a hint of tension and irritation in my voice. The technician does not speak English fluently and asks me to repeat slowly and clearly all the serial numbers and error messages. I am transferred through a progression of other departments, each time repeating all the information I had previously given. As my negativity and frustration build, I remember to breathe and relax, and the tightness I am feeling in my voice releases. I might let out a little humming as I am placed on hold. It feels good to make sound easily. The experience is unpleasant and, if I allow it, my internal struggle will be felt in my voice. The listeners are clueless about my struggle, so that is a blessing.

As a speech therapist, I use my voice extensively for my profession, typically beginning as soon as I wake up and not stopping until late in the evening. With the majority of my clients, I carry the conversational load. Extensive explanations, prompts, and encouraging dialogues are necessary. Add to that the unending phone calls and socially active evenings, and I am pretty much talking most of my waking hours.

There was a time not long ago when none of this was possible. My voice was held hostage by a rare disorder called "spasmodic dysphonia", or SD. Then (2004), I would awake with a sense of dread over my workday, although I had relinquished phone duties and kept my talking to a minimum. I was embarrassed over how dreadful I sounded, and trying to explain it to others made matters worse. I would, by sheer power of will, croak through the day, primarily treating young children who are very forgiving of bad voices. That was the easiest part of my day, but it still took considerable effort on my part. When previously I would chat about how the parents might help with homework assignments and answer their questions, I had to provide written instructions instead. I resorted to a lot of emails.

If the phone rang or colleagues asked for advice, I panicked. Such was the fear I experienced in my mind and body. My stomach would knot up, my breathing would become shallow, and I could barely reply. After six months of living this nightmare, I surrendered, and resigned from my job with the intention of somehow finding a way out of the living hell that was SD.

Free to Speak: Overcoming Spasmodic Dysphonia ©2005

I self-published my first book approximately one year after being diagnosed with SD. It is a 70-page booklet outlining my personal experience and how I was able to come through a very serious and handicapping condition with a fully functioning and essentially normal voice. That book is the story of a woman full of hope, grace, gratitude, and passion. It proposes an outline of voice rehabilitation and an appendix of exercises to guide those with SD, possibly with their therapists, to gain control over lost voices. The purpose of the first book was to provide a commentary of my experience with SD, how I overcame it, and to propose that it was quite possible for others to do the same. I believe the story of the onset of my SD and my journey through it provides valuable insight. It would make an excellent introduction to this book, which provides the proof and a more in-depth examination of the process of voice rehabilitation.

Free to Speak II has been much more difficult to write. I don't know if this is because I have learned too much or not enough. Perhaps it's a bit of both. I fear I cannot adequately put into words what I want to accomplish. I keep up with the research, and there is always something new on the horizon. There are so many unanswered questions about the neurological aspects of voice production. Recent functional Magnetic Resonance Imaging (fMRI) brain studies identified brain activity differences between people with SD and people without SD. I am not surprised or bothered by that information. Voice professionals have been frustrated by the failures of current treatments to manage or cure this condition. While botulinum toxin (Botox®) injections have been the gold standard since the 1980s, we know this is not enough. A comment by the keynote speaker at the 2010 Foundation Voice Symposium clearly expressed our dilemma. "We will never cure SD treating it with Botox. The voice becomes more fluent, but it is weak, and they cannot sing."

My personal theory of how we can manage to overcome a neurological disorder such as SD is that our brains have been shown to create new patterns of activity throughout our lifetimes. A seasoned researcher in the neurological aspects of voice production, Christy Ludlow, PhD, made this statement at the Symposium to conclude her talk about SD, "Neuroplasticity of the brain is the good news." She gave no further suggestions as to how this might work, but at least she acknowledged it. To me, this means finding a new groove, working around the faulty signals to find a new voice. My voice may not be perfect on a day-to-day basis, but it can be very *strong*, and I can sing! How and why? My brain has changed and I produce voice in a new groove. I produce voice in a different way and, therefore, I have created new pathways for voice in my brain. I have no proof, but I believe this is what has happened.

Rules, guidelines, and especially gold standards are never meant to stagnate, especially in the health field. "Challenge of current paradigms" was also a focus of this year's Voice Symposium. How fitting, I thought! I have always loved being a speech pathologist. I have enjoyed reading, researching, journaling, and writing. This book has not come easily *because* it is no longer just "Connie's story." I empathize with the agony in which people with SD often live. I'm angry with the advice they are given and how they are presented such a hopeless outlook day after day, year after year. I want our profession to offer more— something to empower people with SD to become free to speak.

I have been overtly and covertly criticized since I published my first book and largely shunned as I tiptoed into the scientific community. I suppose that is to be expected, for I challenge an established gold standard that makes most professionals feel confident and comfortable. There appears to be a common misperception that my intention is to disprove Botox as a valid treatment for SD. That is not my intention. I believe there are situations in which those with SD will either choose or require this treatment. However, I have discovered another way, one that is more natural and long lasting than Botox, to manage the condition successfully. I believe that this option should be further explored and truthfully offered as an alternative. Stories of successful voice recovery need to be shared. Instead, I and my successful patients are blocked from posting on the forum run by the National Spasmodic Dysphonia Association. I hear story after story of voice professionals diagnosing SD and telling their clients to steer clear of my program because it would be a waste of their time and money. Those who seek out my program without their doctors' approval are consistently glad they did so.

Against criticism a man can neither protest nor defend himself; he must act in spite of it, and then it will gradually yield to him.—Johann Wolfgang von Goethe

A Little History and Defining Moments

Beginning in May 2004 until around January 2005, I was suffering from severe adductor spasmodic dysphonia with tremor. My voice, something I had taken for granted for as many of my 44 years as I could remember, had left me. I sounded as if I were being strangled as I spoke. I fought against that diagnosis and refused to let it cripple me for life. Specialists told me that the condition was incurable and that it would only get worse. They told me that voice therapy would not help and that the gold standard of treatment, botulinum toxin injections, would give me temporary relief. They told me I would most likely need regular injections for the remainder of my life. Apparently, the tremor in my voice indicated that it was a neurological condition. I was not one of the lucky ones who had a psychogenic conversion or muscle tension variety that could be fixed right up with psychological or voice therapy or both.

We all have defining moments in our lives that change who we are. My SD experience was life altering: the journey of a voice lost, the feelings of despair and dire consequences that resulted, and the eventual recovery of freedom in communication. It is a story that I am happy to share over and again as it instills hope and direction to those suffering with this disorder. It is a large part of who I am as a human being and of what I have to contribute to improving the human condition. As we move through our lives, we all have the opportunity to leave the world a better place. I believe my work through SD is one of the major life events that will allow me to do that. There is a purpose in my passion, and there are many people with a need I can relate to through my experience.

As my SD progressed in the early months, it became clear that I needed to devote myself fully to the process of recovery. Back then I had the luxury, if you will, of simply working on my voice and my book. My son was away at college, my daughter was in her senior year of high school, and I had taken a sabbatical from practicing as a speech therapist because of my voice problems. With a kitten in my lap, a dog at my feet, and a cup of tea, I alternated between my voice and breathing exercises, research, and writing. I walked frequently in nature, practiced yoga, meditated, and researched. I prayed a lot. My husband was supportive, financially and emotionally, and we were both ecstatic as my voice slowly returned.

Living with SD was a dark place that was both frightening and frustrating. I felt vulnerable, alone, limited, anxious, and uncertain as to how to navigate my life. After overcoming SD, life became like "sunshine on a cloudy day." I was excited about developing my own business, publishing a book, and watching it consistently sell. I was remaining free to speak in all situations and experiencing success in treating those with SD. I have friends from many countries as a result of my work and have had the opportunity to debate and collaborate with some of the finest voice specialists and related professionals worldwide. While many voice specialists have been skeptical of my work and criticized it rudely, others are accepting and excited about it, especially when they see me and hear me speaking now and hear the audio files of my voice as it was in 2004. My circle of friends, my positive influence in the lives of others, and my world expanded. My confidence grew and I was living in the proverbial bubble of good favor. I was savoring life with much gratitude. There were a few bumps and bruises, but I persevered.

In the process, I was committed to sharing hope with others afflicted with this disorder and to discovering ways to use my experience as a speech pathologist to develop ways to rehabilitate the SD voice. Despite cautions and criticisms from well-meaning professionals that I was promoting a treatment that had not been scientifically proven, I *had* to share my experience. Recovering my voice instilled in me a passion to help others find a way out of the depths of despair resulting from serious voice dysfunction. I was encouraged and supported by the team that had helped me through my journey. If fear crept in, they encouraged me and helped me move into a place of power. I was thankful for the personal growth this opportunity continued to present.

I felt that SD was so complex that it would require a multidisciplinary approach or at least a very intensive holistic methodology. I knew in my heart that what I was offering could not potentially harm anyone. I selected a team of professionals who had been a part of my healing process, including my breathing coach and personal psychologist. The methods I used were already in place in standard voice or stuttering therapy.

Our psychologist used standardized instruments and solid counseling techniques. The breathing specialist, Mike White, had spent twenty-five years researching breathing and had published books and instructional DVDs. We may have all been a bit lacking in SD treatment experience, but we were willing and ready. Although speech therapists are encouraged to utilize only scientifically proven treatments, there are clearly many eclectic approaches to therapy that do not have scientific studies to back them up. I had been my own research experiment, and believed that others could be successful with this method. In August 2005, we launched the first "Free to Speak Holistic Voice Rehabilitation Clinic."

In my life experience, I have found that "wounded healers" are the best kind to have on your side. People were drawn to the clinic primarily because they knew I had experienced successful resolution of SD and that I understood the pain and the process. The many successes over the next several years were evidence that the program really worked.

Sunshine, Shadows, Storms, and Rainbows

Life, however, progresses as a series of highs and lows for all of us. We can't live in the bubble forever and not realize there may come a time that it will burst. My bubble burst in May 2007, when our 21-year-old son was killed in a motorcycle accident near our home. It was in the wee hours of the morning after Mother's Day. As if being hit by a sudden rogue wave, my life changed again. Here was yet another cruel defining moment, unpredicted, unthinkable, and utterly tragic. It was in the second year of the voice clinics. The loss was great, and it still haunts me. But even within this, I was determined to grow into a better person through the pain.

In shock, I moved through the motions. Months earlier, my husband and I had planned a trip to London and Ireland that was scheduled for two weeks after our son's death. We decided it would be best if we could arrange to have our daughter, then nineteen, come along. I even saw clients and gave a talk to the Dystonia Society on that trip. Despite my grief and pain, my voice remained strong. Business was booming and we had so much interest in the clinics that two were held that summer. Perhaps God knew in His infinite wisdom that a busy mind and purposeful actions offered some protection in my fragile state.

My mother-in-law suddenly became ill and passed away at age sixty-nine, just six months after Taylor's death. We were able to spend precious time with her as the cancer destroyed her body and say our goodbyes. Despite losing two precious loved ones in such a short time, my voice seemed unaffected until the shock wore off and the various stages of grief set in. I recall viewing videos in which I was working with SD clients, and my eyes would turn toward our family photo or Taylor's memorial photo. I recall the pain, but yet I appeared unfazed. I performed as a therapist should, and my voice was clear and my instructions strong. People kept recovering their voices. They gave me the privilege of sharing memories and my grief over losing a son and a "mom." Those who had experienced similar losses shared their tears with mine.

Once the shock wore off, there were times of great despair. Through these valleys, there were times it felt very difficult to speak. I learned a lot as I resolved not to let my emotions take my voice hostage. Interestingly, I noted that in my Bereaved Parents meetings, sometimes moms or dads were so overcome by their grief they were literally unable to speak. As it came their turn to tell their stories, they would just pass, speechless. One father called this "grief spasms."

In the second year of bereavement, I spiraled into depression and was stuck there for a time. I also had a few bouts of laryngitis that were frightening because the onset of my SD came after a bout of laryngitis. Yet I never plunged back into the out-of-control strangled voice I had years before. The rainbows always came after the storms. My voice grew stronger and my confidence as well. Eventually the depression lifted with the help of counseling and temporary medication.

I believe that all things happen for a reason, even if we cannot comprehend them at the time. In all hardships, there is opportunity for positive growth. For me, SD was an opportunity for growth, and going back to SD was not an option. I control my voice; it does not control me. This is what I believe and this is what I teach because I feel that God has given all of us a body mind that is never stagnant. Our brain has unlimited potential for change and healing if we seek to access it. I also believe that we are all given a set of life circumstances. In the dark times, we can choose to grow with grace or we can fall victim to our weakness and give up our personal power. As hard as it has been, Taylor's death has given me opportunity for growth. Sharing my experience with others who know that I truly understand what they have been going through is part of the healing for both my personal and professional life.

My desire is to continue to live from my heart and share my experiences, according to God's plan for my life. The purpose of this book is to report preliminary efficacy data, present case studies, and describe the basics of voice rehabilitation. Finally, I have some theories around neuroplasticity that may be relevant in reversing an "incurable" condition or at least finding a new groove for voice production in the brain.

For I know the plans I have for you...plans for a hope and a future.—Jeremiah 29:11, NIV Bible

Chapter 1

Current Medical Views and Research on Spasmodic Dysphonia

Definition of SD

Many readers of this book have already done some preliminary research on spasmodic dysphonia. Most have been informed of the current popular view by one or more doctors or speech therapists. A complete history of the disorder is in my original book as well as most current texts. For the most current professional definition, reference the American Speech-Language-Hearing Association website, www.asha.org, or the National Institute on Deafness and other Communication Disorders, www.nidcd.nih.gov. Simply, it is considered to be a focal dystonia of the laryngeal muscles (those involved in speaking), which seems to affect, primarily, voice production while speaking, less often in singing, and rarely in primary functions such as coughing, grunting, sighing, laughing, or crying. There seems to be a lack of coordination in the many muscles of the larynx and vocal folds during speech.

Although more common in women, with the average age at diagnosis between thirty and fifty years, it occurs in both genders, in teenagers, and in seniors of eighty years and older. Adductor type (AD/SD) is the most prevalent, with over adduction or forceful closure of the vocal folds. Abductor type (AB/SD) is much less common and more difficult to treat. The vocal folds either spasm in the closed position, causing a pressed, strangled voice with breaks (AD/SD), or in the open position, causing extreme breathiness, weak voice, or breathy breaks in the voice (AB/SD). Some people have symptoms of both, at times with a quivering tremor.

According to the National Institute of Health, SD is a rare disease. Incidence and prevalence data vary widely, with lowest estimates at .02 percent of the population, to as many as 70,000 cases in the United States alone. Even this may be an underestimate, according to other sources.

Etiology

Etiology (cause) of SD remains controversial, but it is currently thought to be an incurable neurological condition. It is most frequently described as being in the family of focal dystonias or movement disorders, which includes spasmodic torticollis (neck), blepharospasm (eyelids), writer's cramp and musician's dystonia (hands). An article in *Brain* by Simonyan et al. (2008), reported brain differences in those with spasmodic dysphonia when compared to control groups. Increased activity in the primary sensorimotor cortex has been observed using fMRI studies during symptomatic voice production (Simonyan and Ludlow 2010). Based on these studies, one could consider the dysfunctional patterns of voice production in SD as resulting from abnormal patterns of brain activity. One could question whether the manner of voice production resulted in brain activity changes or vice versa. The somatic and psychological aspects of SD are also presumed to be a result rather than possible cause of the disorder. There are ample unanswered questions at this stage, and the condition can sometimes wax and wane with periods of normal voicing, sometimes described as episodic SD. People sometimes report being cured after a single Botox shot, which is impossible considering how the treatment works. Others go into remission for many years, possibly permanently, and still others are helped with voice therapy.

Botulinum Toxin Treatment

Dr. Andrew Blitzer et al. (1998) is one of the most commonly referenced Ear, Nose and Throat physicians, and is credited with promoting Botox® (Allergan, Inc.) treatment as the gold standard through his initial study of 900 patients over 12 years. His conclusion was that SD is a focal dystonia of neurological origin, characterized by abnormal laryngeal muscle spasms that occur as phonation begins. Treatment with Botox clearly induces a temporary paresis or weakness of laryngeal muscles, which provides short-term relief of symptoms. Repeated injections, generally every three to four months, are required for relief. There is typically a period of aphonia or breathiness, a plateau of good voice production, and then a return of symptoms requiring additional injections. Results seem to vary greatly from one patient to the next, even with different injections by the same doctor. A study by Langeveld et al. (2001) stated that improvement in vocal function has been reported after injections of Botox injections, though a completely normal voice is rarely achieved.

There are other concerns about this treatment. A Cochrane review of the effectiveness of botulinum toxin treatment for SD conducted by Watts, Whurr, and Nye (2006), concluded an inability to draw unbiased generalized conclusions regarding effectiveness for spasmodic dysphonia. A similar meta-analysis by Boutsen et al. (2002) concluded that Botox is only moderately and temporarily effective, and other treatment options should continue to be explored.

Two of the most current articles on the effectiveness of Botox were published in 2010. The first, written by Dr. Blitzer, examines 1300 patients over twenty-four years. His patients included people with adductor, abductor, mixed, and singer's dysphonia. He concluded that 25 percent of those receiving Botox injections had undesirable side effects. For the largest percentage of patients, those with AD/SD, he reported an average of 90 percent of normal function attained for a mean duration of fifteen weeks. For AB/SD patients, an average of 70 percent of normal function was attained for a mean of ten weeks. Singers did not do well with Botox treatment because it decreased loudness and vibrato, and it truncated pitch. Dr. Blitzer did not describe how the percentage of improvement was determined. He also disclosed a conflict of interest; he had received research funding from Allergan and other pharmaceutical companies as well as consultancy fees (Blitzer 2010).

The second study came from the United Kingdom as a retrospective study of Dysport®, manufactured by Ipsen, which is the botulinum toxin product used there in SD patients. It is a commercial botulinum toxin A product equivalent to Botox. The study was based on the authors' experience in treating patients at the Royal National Throat, Nose and Ear Hospital in London, UK. (Behrad *et al.* 2010). A total of sixty-eight patients were identified, all with adductor SD and having had five or more injections. The patients themselves judged the success of a total of 272 injections using a self-reported Voice Score. The authors reported that 94 percent of the injections were successful. Patients rated their best vocal quality after the injection. All scores of 2 (slight improvement) or higher were counted as successful. A score of 3 was a moderate improvement, 4 was marked improvement, and 5 was extreme improvement or nearly normal. The researchers did not report an average percent of improvement or average Voice Score. They reported side effects lasting longer than 2 weeks in 5 percent of patients. No objective voice-related quality of life scores, such as the Voice Handicap Index or the Voice Related Quality Of Life, were included in either this or Blitzer's study.Recently, the Federal Drug Administration issued a Black Box warning for the use of Botox, which is the strongest warning required of a pharmaceutical product. This indicates that botulinum toxin products can cause serious health problems. At this time, injection into the vocal folds is not yet an approved use of the drug, according to the FDA. Allergan was recently fined by the federal government for promoting Botox for conditions for which it has not been approved. Visit the FDA website listed in the bibliography for the full Botox warning. Despite these obvious problems and limitations, botulinum toxin is the most frequently prescribed treatment when SD is diagnosed and, to date, the gold standard. This book is *not* intended to disprove or discredit Botox as a valid treatment, but to offer the personal experience of the writer and her patients. This book presents an alternative method of voice rehabilitation that may be more permanent and satisfactory in relieving the symptoms of SD. Voice rehabilitation may be the first choice for people with SD, or it may be the solution for those who do not get satisfactory relief using Botox.

Other Considerations in SD Treatment

An article by Braden et al. (2010), seeking to determine the effectiveness of Botox treatment for AD/SD, cited that in recent years, more emphasis has been placed on measuring the patient's perception of the impact on quality of life rather than just physical change in the voice. The World Health Organization (WHO) has endorsed this shift to determine the impact of the disease on the whole person. Many speech therapists will attest that SD has dire implications with quality of life issues. Even many people successfully treated with Botox injections continue to feel handicapped and anxious about their condition. The Voice Handicap Index (VHI) is a standardized test that qualifies the level of handicap on three levels: functional, emotional, and perceptual (Jacobson et al. 1997). Patients rate their perception of the impact of their voices on their lives. People with SD consistently have the highest VHI scores of all disorders of the voice (Hy Li et al. 2009).

Voice therapy is gaining in popularity, but only as an adjunct to Botox or as a short-term trial prior to Botox treatment. Research indicates that speech therapy can prolong the benefits of Botox injections (Murray and Woodson 1994). In some cases, voice therapy or coaching has been credited with permanent relief from the disorder (Stemple 2000). In *The Voice Book*, DeVore and Cookman (2009) describe a woman who sought their help after severe hoarseness for nine years and a diagnosis of SD. Treatment with Botox had been recommended, but the therapists determined that her problem was due to chronic tension in the laryngeal muscles and were able to help her regain a normal voice with short-term therapy. Success with voice therapy is found throughout the literature; however, the current view is that it has a poor track record.

Another article by Haselden et al. (2009) examines locus of control in SD and other voice disorders. Locus of control refers to people's perception of being in control and whether they believe they have an influence over their own health or if they give that control to *chance* or *powerful others*. High levels of *internal* control appear to lead to better outcomes in recovery in non-voice health studies. Therefore, the authors applied these variables to those with SD and functional dysphonia. People who believe that they have control over their health receive positive behavioral and psychological results. Those who believe they do not have control may be in a state of "learned helplessness" and do not cope as well.

Perception of control was very different for these two groups, with SD patients having significantly less *internal* control. Those with functional dysphonia were given a positive prognosis and were in a voice therapy program, providing them with a renewed sense of control over their voices. SD patients were receiving Botox treatments, clearly giving over control to an outside source. One comment stuck with me, "Low *internality* could also be a reflection of a sense of hopelessness in the face of an incurable neurological disease." I have seen a shift in this aspect of control in my own patients. When given examples of those who have been able to improve their voices, and a clear plan of treatment, renewed hope results in better control in the vast majority. Perceived helplessness is replaced with hope and direction and better voices!

Even before reading Haselden's article, I was convinced that it was crucial for our patients to have hope and take personal responsibility for getting better. After reading my book and meeting me, patients almost always had a huge shift in their belief systems. I provided a questionnaire for those enrolling in the clinic, which helped them to examine their commitment to the process of voice rehabilitation before they arrived at the clinic. I questioned how important voice recovery was to them and how firmly they believed they could make changes in their lives to accomplish this. I asked them to imagine how their lives could change if their voices improved. Throughout the clinic experience, self-exploration and responsibility were key topics.

People with SD do not need a therapist just saying, "Do this or that exercise two times daily for six weeks." Standard treatments for SD do not sufficiently address the issue that the problem requires self-exploration and personal responsibility beyond a set of exercises, or that rehabilitation may be a lengthy process. Additionally, voice therapists are taught that therapy is unlikely to be of much benefit. Botox, of course, gives full responsibility to the physician administering the drug. Voice therapy sessions are typically short-term and do not sufficiently teach people to look at their problems holistically. Self-responsibility for overall health, fitness, stress management, psychological well-being, and examination of belief systems about change are rarely addressed.

Botulinum toxin still remains the most frequently prescribed treatment for people diagnosed with SD. It certainly has its rightful place, but I hope the paradigm will shift with the recent interest in quality of life and locus of control issues. In our attempts to treat patients with dignity and respect and, above all, to "do no harm" as our Hippocratic Oath dictates, we need to help patients gain better control over their voices. If we tell them they must rely only on Botox for relief, we render them crippled.

My diagnosing speech pathologist, a specialist in the field of voice, thought her professional duty was to provide me with a proper diagnosis and counsel me on what that meant. In her opinion, SD would continue to worsen, voice therapy would be slightly helpful in masking my symptoms at best, and what I needed was a Botox shot as soon as possible. I chose a different way, or I might be giving over my control to Botox injections today. People continue to come through my door and tell me how they, too, were given no hope or alternative to Botox. It is wonderful to report that many of them have proven that a valid alternative exists.

Surgical Options

Surgical procedures for SD have also increased recently. The most common procedure in the United States is selective laryngeal adductor denervation-reinnervation (SLAD/R) surgery, described by Dr. Gerald Burke in 1999. A study of the long-term results (2006) involving eighty-three patients with an average follow-up of four years indicated significantly improved Voice Handicap Index scores in 83 percent of patients, with 91 percent agreeing that their voices were more fluent after the surgery. Perceptual evaluation of the voices indicated voice breaks in 26 percent and breathiness in 30 percent. I also have heard personal accounts of people who feel that their voice is about 95 percent normal several years after the surgery. Outside the study, I have received personal accounts of complete failure to produce any improvement post-surgically as well as ongoing problems such as permanent loss of voice or eventual return of symptoms over a period of months or years. Some patients have needed additional surgical procedures or have continued Botox injections following the surgery. As with any major surgery, risks need to be carefully evaluated and compared with potential benefit. Medicare now covers this surgery, making it an easier option for seniors, but risks still should be explicitly explained.

Another common surgery for abductor SD is vocal fold medialization surgery, in which stents are inserted to bring the vocal cords closer together. I have seen clients who elected this option but have not heard a completely normal voice as a result. Compensatory behaviors can be unraveled and voice improved with therapy. Currently, most doctors agree that surgery should be a final option after all other possibilities for treatment have been explored.

Chapter 2
Alternatives to the Mainstream View of SD

There are many promises of cures for SD, from acupuncture, drugs, herbal remedies, homeopathic solutions, laser therapy, osteopathy, and chiropractic adjustments, to just about any alternative path imaginable. All of these have promise in helping many conditions. Most are anecdotal case studies with few patients, but they are found in the literature. I do not recommend any of these treatments as a cure for SD, but I do not discourage them. They are non-invasive and may help some aspects of the voice dysfunction. I would only suggest that people not give over their personal power and responsibility to any of these professions or methods but rather view them as part of the holistic approach likely to result in lasting change, which I believe to be an internal process.

Morton Cooper's DVR

Any discussion of spasmodic dysphonia treatment would be incomplete without a discussion of Direct Voice Rehabilitation (DVR) as described by speech pathologist Morton Cooper, PhD in the 1970s. It is my intention to be honorable to the contributions Dr. Cooper has made with regard to viewing SD as curable, but also to present my interpretation of his approach based on personal experience and reports from his previous patients. He has written several books, most recently *Curing*

Hopeless Voices: The Strangled Voice (Spasmodic Dysphonia) & Other Voice Problems with Direct Voice Rehabilitation (2006). When first diagnosed, I read Dr. Cooper's material, specifically *Change Your Voice, Change Your Life* (1984). I was presented with few options for voice improvement and none for recovery, and I simply could not accept the information as it was presented to me. When I inquired about Dr. Cooper, I was told that he was not respected and was considered a "quack" by most professionals. I was told that he gave false hope to desperate people and that to visit him would be a waste of time and money. However, I found hope in his book and tape and some improvement in my voice with his suggested simple exercises. I knew that there were people who had recovered their voices with his program.

Seeking Dr. Cooper's Cure

I contacted Dr. Cooper because no one else could give me any hope. He told me that I needed to come to California for at least two weeks, which was very expensive. I explained that I was a speech therapist myself and I just needed some guidance. He told me he would not see me for less than a complete week. I had to convince him to see me for an initial consultation and maybe a day of therapy.

I asked for a visit to Dr. Cooper as a gift for my forty-fifth birthday, which I felt was my best chance to escape from the prison of SD. My mother and my husband came together to make it happen. Just three months after onset and one month after diagnosis, I set off for Los Angeles. It was with great anticipation that I embarked on this adventure. I arrived at Dr. Cooper's office, which, interestingly, was like a step back into the 1970s. He greeted me and began immediately to assess my condition by asking some questions and listening to me talk. He told me that I had severe SD, but that I could recover my voice. He used his "instant voice press", quick jabs with his fingers into my solar plexus as I was saying "ah", to assess my pitch. He instructed me to speak in a higher pitch, and when I did so, my voice became clearer. I beamed happily—my voice was returning. He told me I was just using my voice incorrectly and that I could definitely recover it. My husband still talks about how my whole demeanor changed that day. I now had *hope*.

Never deprive someone of hope; it might be all they have.—H. Jackson Brown, Jr.

Peer Support

Dr. Cooper soon asked if I wanted to meet a few others with my condition. Of course, I did! I met a lady who also had AD/SD, and we practiced in a room with a machine called the Voice Mirror, which showed us our pitch targets. We mostly just practiced on our own, with Dr. Cooper occasionally checking in with us to tell us to speak higher. Most of the time, he was quietly typing on a typewriter in the adjoining office. It was rather surreal, but we experienced freedom of speech together that day, gazing at the lights on the Voice Mirror that cued us if our pitch dropped too low. I asked for help with breathing, and he gave me some rudimentary instruction: "Lie down and put your hand on your stomach. Breathe in and your stomach should go out. Vocalize and it should go in." My primary teacher over those two days was my practice partner. She sounded great, and she told me her voice had been worse than mine but that she had been practicing for almost a week.

Most people with SD have *never* met another person with the disorder. That is a lonely feeling. It was very freeing and empowering to meet someone who shared the experience of SD and was talking better than I was. I was hearing fairly normal voices telling me they used to be worse than me. I saw videos of people that Dr. Cooper had "cured". In my inner being, I grabbed that power and declared that I would no longer be controlled by this disorder. I was ready to claim personal power for changing my voice. I also had faith that God would grant me His grace and power and that in His perfect time, I would speak again.

Morton Cooper had the courage to approach SD in an innovative way and paved the way for what I do today in the area of voice rehabilitation. I believe we both see value in the ability to recover the voice when one is diagnosed with SD, and the value of peer support in the process. Because our approaches to treatment are vastly different, however, they need no comparison.

Holistic Intensive Voice Rehabilitation

Unfortunately, as soon as my first book was published, I was viewed with extreme skepticism in the professional world of SD. Was I trying to follow in Dr. Cooper's footsteps? Did I receive a misdiagnosis? Was I preying on desperate people to make a fast buck? Was I simply in a temporary remission? I felt the virtual breath-holding of the professional community, the attempts to avoid me at meetings, the fake niceness. I was banned from posting on the National Spasmodic Dysphonia Association (NSDA) online support forum, and my clients were banned from mentioning their successes with the clinic or my name as someone who had helped them. There were some very nasty accusatory posts that were potentially harmful to my reputation.

I had the best of intentions and my aim was to help people and present new information, yet I was attacked. I fought for fair treatment in that arena, writing letters to both NSDA and ASHA for about a year until I grew weary of the fight. Allegan, the drug company that produces Botox, funds the NSDA website as well as most of the research for SD. I was not going to get anywhere, and it was a waste of my time. Although their refusal to post successes from my patients were explained away as "blocked because they appear to be advertising," there were ample posts about specific doctors and clinics providing Botox injections and discussions of the results of surgical procedures. I saw no purpose in fighting the establishment. I retreated, and I very rarely visit the website because it feels healthier to accept the situation as it is and just know that those who need our approach will find it.

The idea for holistic intensive voice rehabilitation was born of my own experience. On my journey to recovery, I sought out the help of various disciplines. First, I knew my breathing was a mess. An online search led me to Michael White, previously a commercial real estate broker who changed careers on his life journey to develop an Optimal Breathing Program. He provided a training program and worked with people with all kinds of breathing disorders. I took his online breathing test and recognized that I had a serious problem with breathing. I ordered his book and DVD and worked with that for a while. I later made a three-hour appointment and experienced his hands-on work. There is nothing like experiencing full, complete breathing when it has been seriously dysfunctional. I realized that my fast, shallow breathing was impeding the foundational support my voice needed. Mike had techniques and breathing development tools so I could continue to work on my own. He helped me discover a strong voice that could ride out on the breath.

I was a mess emotionally. I had experienced great stress in the year prior to the onset of SD, and psychological counseling was a key element for me. Initially, I learned ways to manage my anxiety and depression. Once SD took over my life, I learned ways to manage the weakness this condition brings and give up my perfectionism. I eventually took a leave from my job, looking for some good to come from this disaster. I learned to recognize how my perceptions could keep me stuck or help me to heal. I learned from my counselor and many self-help books that I could be an active partner in healing my body by using my mind and my spiritual connection to God.

My body was extremely tense and out of balance. I began regular massage and yoga and studied the technique of F.M. Alexander, which deals with postural adjustments aimed at optimizing the functions of the body, including the voice. This technique aims to inhibit tensions and postures that interfere, and develop awareness of proper form and function. It took time, but my body began to open up and relax, and I came to see how body postures and bad habits restricted my breathing and my voice. Some of my bad habits came through the experiences of my lifetime, and others as compensations for my SD. As I increased my effort in trying to speak, the compensations worsened and my body became more tightly wound internally.

In my quest for voice recovery, I tried all the voice therapy techniques I had studied. These included trying resonant voice techniques (Verdolini 2005), finding optimal pitch, managing all the subsystems of voice production, and singing. I tried it all, keeping what worked for me and eliminating what did not. Confidential voice, or using a very quiet voice just above a whisper, worked well to help me decrease my effort. Learning to speak calmly while in the middle of the storm within my mind body was critical. I experimented on myself, tried to be playful with my voice, recovered my voice, and wrote my book.

"Holistic intensive" is possibly the most appropriate description of what can help people with SD. Since it is a rare disorder, and one that other people seldom understand, I believe that it is most worthwhile to bring together people to a common place to learn and recover together. The breathing and psychological pieces to recovery are priceless. I have treated those with SD individually with success, yet I still prefer the clinics. There is a depth there that cannot be replicated in individual sessions.

I truly believed that those who I could help would find me, and that seems to be the case today. As I take on a more relaxed approach, the clinics seem to happen with minimal advertising and almost no criticism. If I tiptoe into the scientific arena, it can become quite stressful and intimidating. The anxiety I feel there is **not** good for my voice. I only occasionally get referrals from voice professions, and sometimes SD patients are cautioned not to buy into this type of treatment. Currently, the idea of rehabilitation of the SD voice is accepted by only a choice few of my fellow professionals, but I hope that in time this will change.

Is There a Cure for SD?

This is the million dollar question! Since the 1970s, when Dr. Cooper declared that he had the cure and that SD was merely a misuse of the voice that he could fix right up with his DVR, this has been the major criticism and challenge. After five years of helping people with SD and experiencing some excellent success stories, I do not think that cure is the word that I would use. I prefer to use recovered or rehabilitated, as SD can be pesky and inconsistent, and a cure would imply no further symptoms ever. In most cases, success with SD is the management of a chronic disorder through a rehabilitation of the voice. To be successful, rehabilitation needs to be holistic and comprehensive. The discovery of a different voice groove can have an amazing impact on voice production and can tease the voice back to normal over time.

I do not believe that SD is simply a result of misuse of the voice, unless that chronic misuse leads to changes in the brain. SD is a neurological condition and I believe that I still have it. I'm not cured, but I am no longer handicapped by my voice. I am free to speak in all situations. I've found a new groove that works for me. I have seen it work for others. No one asks me if I am sick or if I am losing my voice. Acoustically, my voice is normal most of the time. At its worst, it is a bit tight and raspy or lacking full resonance, but so are most voices on occasion.

I am a work in progress and a living example that SD can be overcome without drugs or surgery. I have not had a Botox injection, so I cannot discuss that experience personally. However, as a result of what we teach at the clinics, a significant number of people have gained better control of their voices and decreased their perceived level of handicap. Voice rehabilitation has no side effects and no risks, and if it can help people recover normal voice production, or even to improve and, therefore, become less handicapped by their voices, it should be included in the discussion of SD treatment. It may take decades for it to become a valid treatment option, but I am committed to promoting it.

Cognitive-Behavioral Approach to Change

SD treatment, the way we have developed it, is a cognitive-behavioral program that aims to change thinking patterns, habits, and behaviors, which have the power to change the brain. I propose that what happens is that the normal groove or sensory-motor neural pathway for voicing has lost its way. These automatic functions of voicing that most of us take for granted cease to work properly. For years, we have opened our mouths to speak our minds, and our voices cooperated. Suddenly, in cases like mine, or over a period of time, the voice stops cooperating. We don't understand what is happening and we panic. It feels all wrong, and we are horrified, self-conscious, and confused. Here starts a struggle that usually is only the beginning of a decline in proper voice production. It feels hard to speak, so we try harder. The harder we try, the worse our voices sound. We may have a good day only to find ourselves literally speechless the next. We go into terrible overcompensations in our efforts to bring our voices under control because we have not had to control them before. These attempts on our part might further disorganize the brain's ability to coordinate the voice.

Other focal dystonias affect the body in similar ways. A professional pianist suddenly can no longer control the movement of certain fingers. This disorganization can be viewed as abnormal activity in the portion of the brain responsible for control of finger movements on brain scans. Correction of the dystonia by physical therapy or rehabilitation can be seen as a change in the activity in the brain. The cause of hand dystonia is theorized as increased sensory input from repetitive practice, which then affects the motor pathway. Could SD be caused by increased sensory input and wrong or repetitive use of the voice? Certainly, we see a lot of patients who use their voices heavily in emotional situations (pastors, attorneys, teachers, real estate brokers, sales representatives, etc.) I have always been a big talker and a perfectionist in my job. In the years before SD, I was not only seeing a high volume of patients, but was also supervising students and clinical fellows, parenting, and volunteering. Did I practice repetitive voice use? Most definitely I did. I talked all day in one capacity or another. I was often trying to control or influence others in the process.

In 1983, Michael Merzenich at the University of California in San Francisco described cortical reorganization after years of studying cortical re-mapping following brain injury or limb amputation. Dr. Jeffrey Swartz then questioned how the brain might remodel itself in response to behavioral demands. They were finding, in studies of monkey brains, that learning and paying attention to new tasks changed the brains. In 1993 at the NIHDS, Alvaro Pascual-Leone reported human studies of neuroplasticity in blind people who read in Braille. Scientists examined string players with six to seventeen years of experience and, comparing them to non-musicians, found that substantial cortical reorganization occurs in the left hand of string players. They also found that *attention* is crucial for use-dependent brain changes. Learning to *pay attention* to how one produces voice is a challenge!

The aforementioned examples are found in *The Mind and the Brain,* by Schwartz and Begley (2002), where they applied these studies to the neurological condition of obsessive-compulsive disorder (OCD). Brain scans paired the condition to faulty neurological activity, which, when treated by a cognitive-behavioral approach, changed along with a reduction in symptoms. We have the ability to do this same thing with SD. The process includes aspects of motor learning and paying attention.

Mind body approaches to healing various medical problems are described by John Sarno, MD (2006). I can relate to this mind body approach for SD. It suggests a psychogenic manifestation, which is certainly evident in some cases of SD. The mind body approach still helps me today when I am in stressful situations and not feeling up to par emotionally. I have to use my mind to process my emotions so they don't take my voice hostage. I have to talk to my brain and convince it that I am in control of my voice. I believe it is critical to understand how intricately the way that we think affects the neurological functioning of our brains. Even in light of the neurological problems we might be encountering, because of faulty neural activity, we can still find control and be responsible for change.

Chapter 3
Keeping SD at Bay

Since my first book outlines my story of overcoming SD, I will not repeat it, but I will continue from the conclusion of the first book and expand on what has happened with my voice since that time. Clarifications from that book as well as expanded viewpoints will follow. I used a holistic approach to recover my voice. It started with hope and belief that it could be done, followed by dedicated re-grooving of the voice and breathing patterns that became automatic for my mind body.

Key ingredients for my success included a right mindset (psychological counseling helped), attention to the mechanics of good voice production (breathing, focus, pitch, and resonance), auditory and visual feedback of the voice, practice, and regaining the feeling of ease or control in voice production. It took approximately eight months to regain a fully functioning voice. While I have had many carefree days with regard to my voice, I still continue to have periodic symptoms, which are mainly perceived only by me. Periodic perceived symptoms can occur with illnesses such as upper respiratory infections or laryngitis, strong emotions, fatigue, anxiety, or allergic reactions. At times, it simply feels more difficult to talk. If you have SD, you understand this feeling of difficulty. If not, it is rather like being very tired or having to speak when you don't have the energy to do so.

Before SD, I rarely felt difficulty speaking, although I had frequent sore throats from early childhood, laryngitis once a year since my teenage years, and a fear of public speaking. Post-SD, I cannot always assess why I feel effort in speaking. However, I do know that I have the tools to speak freely. I know to ignore the effort and just communicate, and my voice will be there for me. It is usually just a few breaths and hums away. I counsel my clients at the stage of recovery when they are experiencing success and others are not commenting on their voice quality, to record and listen often to their voices. It may be necessary to convince themselves the voice sounds better than it feels when there is an internal struggle. It helps to act as if one doesn't have a voice problem because others often don't notice it anyway. I find that listeners react more to one's body posture, facial expressions, and the degree of struggle they manifest outwardly than to the actual sound of the voice. The greater one struggles with the voice, the worse the symptoms become.

I no longer "practice" using my voice, except that daily I attend to it as needed. If it feels difficult, I know to adjust the focus of my voice upward into the face, maybe hum a little to get there, release any tension in the solar plexus, open my shoulders and chest, and breathe properly, allowing my diaphragm to extend downward. I then lift and lighten the voice a bit. I feel that with every adjustment, I am developing a new, easier groove for my voice. I believe this is happening in my brain, literally. At the onset of SD, I found it difficult to hum, sing, or speak. I had voice breaks and times when no voice came. People always asked me about my voice. Now it is consistently easy to hum and sing, and only difficult to speak in specific situations and, even then, just temporarily. I do maintain a regular exercise routine of walking outdoors and practicing yoga. I try to hum and sing frequently throughout the day, throwing in a few glides or trills to stay loose. I attempt to simply communicate and not think too much about how I am producing voice. It then flows more freely, and I am always able to speak.

Viewing SD from a Holistic Perspective

I have come to view SD as more of a holistic issue than I first imagined: that the mind and body are linked intimately, and what the mind dictates, the body follows. Cortical re-mapping and neuroplasticity are proven. All of the research in this area has served to strengthen this view. Zuener et al. (2008) described how writer's cramp (a focal hand dystonia) could be improved or corrected using either task-specific or non-task specific exercises. The important issue was reorganizing the disorganization in the sensory-motor cortex that occurs with this disorder. This reorganization is possible, and I believe that in time, SD will be just a memory for me, not an experience. Time proves this. With every day that I am completely free to speak, even if it feels hard, I am living proof that it is possible to beat this disorder, to re-groove voice production in the brain.

I have learned invaluable lessons from every SD sufferer with whom I've worked. I learned from my own recovery, but learned even more after working with more than one hundred people diagnosed with SD. Naturally, there are still many unanswered questions. Why is it so easy for some people to shift over to a new voice while others seem to try so hard and never attain it? Why does it take some people a week and others many years to attain a good voice? Why do some try so hard to take a natural approach but finally resign themselves to Botox or surgery while others spend years depending on medical remedies before moving to alternatives that work? Why do some absolutely buy into the medical model without considering that they might be able to break free of SD naturally if they desire to? After relying on the medical model for twenty years or more, some are then successful with our approach. No case of SD is just like another, which is what makes this mysterious disorder so difficult to treat. Every person must be analyzed and treated as an individual, though the diagnosis may be the same.

Attempting to put together a program to treat SD is frustrating. It is agonizing to communicate with other speech pathologists and not be able to tell them what to do with their patients because I have not heard their patients speak, felt them breathe, and discussed their emotions or lifestyles with them. I try to explain that voice therapy several times a week is unlikely to help a person with SD and that it is a life change, not just a voice change that has to occur. I also ponder if there is a way to determine who would be best suited to a voice rehabilitation program. I've frequently discussed this with Renata Whurr, PhD, a voice specialist in London with many years of experience in treating SD, largely with the medical model (botulinum toxin injections), but also behaviorally with some success. We agree that some people are not going to be able to take their condition into their own hands. Some people come in with serious emotional issues such as clinical depression or post-traumatic stress syndrome that must be addressed before the voice problems can be dealt with. There are medical problems such as vocal fold paralysis or muscle tension dysphonia misdiagnosed as SD. There may be cases of SD in which the off-groove malfunction of brain activity is stubbornly unable to respond to attempts to change it. There are those that, for various reasons, are not going to comply with a cognitive-behavioral program.

I know enough to realize I am not even close to having all the answers. I know with every cell of my being that SD can be overcome. Voices can be recovered. I see it and hear it, and the stories keep me working. It is not important for me to become famous or for the professional community to recognize me. However, every person who overcomes SD and becomes free to speak is a hero to me, and they are the ones who keep me going. My ultimate goal would be to change the current world paradigm around our thinking about SD. SD should be viewed in a class of serious voice dysfunctions, many of which, although functionally neurological in origin, could be re-grooved using a cognitive-behavioral approach. I believe all newly diagnosed patients should be given access to intensive voice rehabilitation reimbursable by insurance companies. We need to spread hope, not hopelessness.

What We Say and Believe Matters!

I hear too many stories of doom and gloom presented to patients diagnosed with SD. While some are grateful that they aren't just crazy and that there is some reason for their voice difficulties, the "incurable" message is damaging. They may be relieved to have a name for their problem and to know that there is a treatment that will give them temporary relief. They are most likely told that voice therapy will not help. Therefore, if they attempt a trial of therapy, which neither they nor their therapists really believe will make much of a difference; it is highly unlikely to help.

In Latin, placebo means "I will please." Placebos have been used in research studies to determine the true effectiveness of certain procedures or drugs. A placebo may be a dummy medication, and if a study is blinded, the person does not know if he or she is receiving the real drug/treatment or the fake. A certain percentage of people will report improvements when given a placebo. I recently read a study of Parkinson's disease in which placebos were very effective. When given a placebo, it actually changed a person's dopamine levels, which is exactly what the body needed. This increase only occurs if the person is told they are taking the real drug. They believe it will help them and, therefore, it does. If it is a fake, nothing more than a sugar pill, how can it help? The mind body is powerful. Thought becomes reality.

The term nocebo, which few people are aware of, is the opposite of placebo. The term nocebo, with regard to medical treatments, was first coined in 1961 by Walter Kennedy. It is the exact opposite of placebo and in Latin means "I shall harm." Kennedy described a nocebo as a subject-centered response to a belief that something may be harmful. The outcome would be totally generated by the subject's negative expectation. Research has shown that the nocebo effect can reverse the body's response to true medical treatment from positive to negative (Root-Bernstein 1998). Because of ethical concerns, nocebos are not commonly used in medical practice or research. However, some studies commonly support the validity of this effect. In one such study, more than 75 percent of thirty-four college students developed headaches when told that a nonexistent electrical current passing through their heads could produce a headache. In the famous Farmington Heart Study, women whose doctors told them that they had high risk factors for heart disease were four times more likely to die as women with similar risks who were not told of them. (Voelker 1996). Consider the implications in terms of successful outcomes for SD. Should doctors tell patients that they can't manage SD without drugs and then expect them to? Should they tell them to try therapy that is unlikely to help and expect it to have positive results?

When I was first diagnosed, I began to research voraciously. The internet is a wonderful tool but can be overwhelming with the amount of information available. I recall reading about dystonias and how there can be a spread of one type to another. I began to be fearful, and my eye began to twitch. I panicked.

Is this blepherospasm? Then my right shoulder began to ache. Oh no, is it torticollis? My right hand cramped, so maybe I was getting writer's cramp, too? It spiraled for the next few days until I realized what my mind was doing to my body! The very suggestion was becoming a reality until I stopped it mentally. Soon, the physical symptoms also disappeared.

I strongly urge our profession to take care what we tell people about SD. The truth is that some do overcome it, and we simply do not understand exactly how and why. We must not abandon hope because we may just be doing someone harm. Remember, that is against our Hippocratic Oath. Do no harm! Believe you can help those with SD speak normally again. Dream it. Do it! Empower them.

Whatever you do, or dream you can, begin it. Boldness had genius and power and magic in it.—Johann Wolfgang Von Goethe

Chapter 4

The Birth of the Intensive Holistic Voice Rehabilitation Clinic

The Intensive Holistic Voice Rehabilitation Clinic was proposed and initiated in August 2005 as a result of my personal recovery from SD. Throughout the process, we have changed and adapted as needed. We expanded the clinic from three and a half days to five days, and we added on some beneficial services that were not in place for the original clinics. In retrospect, the length of the clinic and the added services, such as lunches together and relaxing massages, have not really changed the outcome significantly. We are constantly re-evaluating the process, and in the future we may move toward empowering people to take control of their own journeys, with educated guidance, which may lead to more small group or seminar-type treatment programs.

Here is how the program currently works. Initially, people find us and inquire about the program, most commonly after searching the internet for spasmodic dysphonia or after reading my book. Initially, the clinic staff consisted of me as administrator and speech pathologist, Michael White as breathing coach, and Robbie Goss as psychologist. In 2007, my daughter, Megan Pike, provided a 45 minute massage for each participant until her university studies took precedence, and Christine Deschler, a talented massage therapist replaced her. Christine also helps with lunches and housekeeping tasks which assist me greatly. She is studying to become a yoga instructor as well so we plan to have her do some yoga introduction/training in the near future. Naturally, evolution in all businesses is necessary at times. Currently Dennis Price from Ft. Lauderdale is serving as our breathing coach. With his extensive life-coaching training with Tony Robbins and his certification as a neurolinguistic programming therapist, he brings a broader perspective. He is also a neuromuscular therapist with extensive knowledge of head and neck anatomy and breathing physiology. He has completed training with Michael White in Optimal Breathing® and is an exciting addition to our team. Mike continues to offer private breathing instruction and Optimal Breathing Schools at his office in Charlotte, North Carolina.

We limit the program to six participants, which is the maximum number we can treat successfully under our current model. Once people enroll in the clinic, they must complete the following documents: the Taylor-Johnson Psychosocial Assessment (online), a case history form, a medical clearance request, a questionnaire about the expectations of the clinic, and the Voice Handicap Index-30.

The first day of the clinic, our clients arrive at noon for a lunch together and to get acquainted and get their materials. We spend the afternoon in assessments and consultations. The psychologist spends time discussing the results of the psychosocial assessment and gives everyone projects to help them strengthen weak social/emotional areas. We conduct breathing and voice assessments, which include acoustic analysis and interviews, concluding with an overview and introductions.

The following days begin with a calm centering exercise and focus on developing breathing, voice, posture, and mind body explorations, either individually or in small groups. We begin at 9 a.m. and continue until late afternoon or early evening. On Saturday night, we have a group dinner and social that includes karaoke (with no pressure to participate). We meet as a group to discuss what is working and try out new skills periodically throughout the week.

The hardest part is assessing individuals and establishing what they need to do to find and begin to groove in the new voice, while teaching them to rely on their own feedback. We work with breathing patterns, which are almost universally unbalanced in SD. All clients are trained in a variety of voice production methods and in use of the Estill Voiceprint program© so they can visualize their pitch and resonance and hear their progress. I find that working on voice image and negative emotional issues is vital for some and not an issue for others. Mechanics can be a huge issue, or one might only need a few adjustments. There are some basics we teach everyone, but certain techniques are more appropriate for adductor SD and others are more helpful for abductor SD. During the week, everyone receives an upper body massage to unravel tensions. Some say this is the first massage they have ever experienced and can see how it could be a helpful part of the plan. The group enjoys healthy lunches together every day and a relaxing waterside view. Our clients freely chitchat with no embarrassment or concern. All improve daily, some in huge leaps and others in small increments.

The last day of the clinic is on Sunday, and it begins with an optional devotion time when people of all religious backgrounds are free to talk about their spiritual journeys and share information that might encourage the others. We also engage in dialogue about the experience of the clinic in the group setting. Each client completes a compliance contract of his or her specific plan, using a holistic model. They are asked to write out goals in the relaxation/fitness, breathing, voice rehabilitation, psychosocial, dietary/nutritional, spiritual, and occupational areas. Connie and Dennis go over the contracts on the final afternoon, and make any needed tweaking of goals. Finally, a reassessment includes a follow-up acoustic analysis and a comparison of the initial voice samples with the improved ones.

Videotaping throughout the week is done during individual voice sessions as well as group interactions. Specific instruction for each person is demonstrated so that when clients leave, they will receive a DVD of their experiences at the clinic as a reminder and a guide of what to do in the coming months or years to maintain the gains and continue to improve. I recently received an email that read, "I just got the DVD of our work together and now, after much laughter, am back to doing my breathing and speaking exercises. What a great tool the video is! I only watched part of it and picked up a lot of practice techniques I had forgotten. You are truly on purpose in your life. I also got a phone call from Mike to see how I was doing. May you both be blessed. Thanks, Connie, for being you."—TM, client.

All clients are asked to complete a program evaluation, which allows us to determine which aspects of the clinic are most beneficial. Clients estimate their percentage of improvement during the clinic and give suggestions about what might make their experience more successful. The program evaluation is also where we get the online testimonials that are posted after each clinic. It seems evident from the feedback that every person with SD participating in the clinic believes it was a valuable experience at the end; this is also maintained by the majority who send in long-term feedback. Even if clients later decide to use Botox treatment, they have many tools with which to work to help strengthen their voices.

Finally, to maximize success, we offer six hours of post-clinic feedback at no additional cost; three hours are with me and three are with Dennis, the breathing coach. It can be by phone, email, or in person. We want to make ourselves accessible when people are having trouble. However, we put a six-month time limit on this offer because some people do not comply with the contract they have developed, and the first six months are so important in the re-establishment of optimal voice production. After that time, if compliance is poor, the clients tend to forget much of what they learned at the clinic. We then ask that clients first review both the DVD and their contracts, and offer consultations for our usual fee. Long-term follow-up is first requested between six and eight months after the clinic. In addition, we invite feedback as long as people will offer it. I send out periodic newsletters by email to those who I have treated, sending encouragement, new research findings, success stories, and always asking for feedback. We learn to maximize the clinic experience as we gather and analyze long-term feedback. The program is definitely evolutionary. We grow and learn from each set of participants, and I also learn from self-exploration and my ongoing research.

Chapter 5
How Well Does the Program Work?— Efficacy Data

It has been easy to collect data. I have boxes of videotapes, standardized test scores, acoustic analysis readings before and after the clinic, and personal testimonials. The problem with determining efficacy with scientific rigor is that our clinic does not follow a specifically definable modality. It is individualized to each person. It is holistic and multi-faceted and takes liberty at teaching and training people to use their own mind bodies to make permanent changes in the way they breathe and use their voices. We aim to change the way they view and use their voices and therefore empower them to make changes that may eventually change their brain patterns. *That* would take a lot of investigating, and it may be impossible to prove just which part of such a multidimensional treatment program helped.

Voice rehabilitation is a different road for each person, and changes may occur quickly or take years. It is a very complex process. Ours is an eclectic approach, which, according to Joseph Stemple, PhD, and author of *Voice Therapy: Clinical Studies* (2002), is a valid approach to use with complex voice disorders. Not only is it valid for SD; it is necessary. At times my approach feels more like an intuitive art process than a scientific one, and perhaps it is. I find myself drawn to the more artistic forms of voice work, such as that of Arthur Lessac (Munro et al. 2009), and the Alexander technique (Heirich 2005), than to the scientific models. I tried them all, it seems, and even at my recent visit to the 2010 Voice Foundation Symposium, the performing arts talks were much fresher and freeing. I found myself doodling on my notepad during some of the scientific presentations: "This information could never help someone with SD."

Efficacy that is controlled for our treatment alone is challenging. Some patients have already been using the program from my book or an Optimal Breathing DVD or both; some have used Botox extensively or had surgeries. Others have improved considerably before attending the clinic through work with a psychologist, speech therapist or their own self-explorations; hence, no pre-treatment tape. People continue to improve years after the clinic, at times difficult or impossible to track because they live in another state or country. Voice samples are needed, yet they are hard to obtain.

In spite of those difficulties, since the current emphasis on SD treatment is on quality of life issues (Haselden et al. 2009), the VHI data we collect is an appropriate and viable method of measuring effectiveness of the program. It is highly sensitive to the perceptions of the client and does not depend on outside ratings. Efficacy is based on self-rating of level of improvement and a standardized instrument (VHI-30). The following is posted on my website.

First Efficacy Study, August 2005—July 2007

There were a total of thirty-eight participants seen in the voice clinic during this period. At 6 months, follow-up data was requested. Thirty responded to the request, with eight lost to follow-up. Each person completed a Voice Handicap Index (VHI) to compare to the initial one they completed before coming to the clinic and a brief questionnaire. Twenty-seven of thirty completed the requested paperwork, with the remaining three sending brief emails. Three participants reported resuming botulinum toxin injections as their treatment of choice 1-8 months following the clinic. One tried Botox once more without success before resuming the program. Two were able to tolerate smaller doses and continue voice exercises. In the three cases where Botox was used primarily as the treatment of choice, VHI scores and questionnaires were not included in efficacy data. This was so that improvements were attributed to using voice rehabilitation without the possible added benefit of botulinum toxin.

A significant decrease in VHI scores was reported in 81% of participants. A change of 18 points on the VHI has been validated to indicate significant change in perceived level of handicap rendered by voice function in three different areas. Average decrease in VHI was calculated for the July group to be 34 points. When asked to rate their level of voice improvement overall, 88% reported moderately to significantly improved voice production. Two people reported slight improvement, and one reported a continued worsening of her voice following the clinic.

The least improvements correlated directly with the degree of compliance to the recommended program. In one case, however, difficulty was attributed to over-effort and subsequent emotional distress. Those who had not complied felt they may need to do so. Clearly, there is a pattern of improvement over time. Follow-up emails up to two years or more often indicate continued improvement in voice ease and production.

Second Efficacy Study, July 2007—August 2008

There were a total of thirty-seven participants seen in the clinic during this period. At 6 months, data was requested and received at 8 months, up to a year later. The VHI -30 was sent, as well as a brief questionnaire, which were the same documents used in the initial study. Twenty-eight of the thirty-seven provided feedback, with 12 lost to follow-up completely, and some sending brief email documentation about how they were progressing. Three participants reported resuming Botox treatments and one had SLAD/R surgery followed by another surgical procedure. As in the first study, those scores were excluded in the efficacy report so that improvement noted here did not reflect improvement in voice production relative to botulinum toxin injections or surgeries.

A significant decrease in VHI scores was reported by 81%, with a range from 0 to105 point decrease. The average decrease was 36 points. When asked to rate their level of improvement, 80% reported moderate to significant improvement in voice production. Four indicated no improvement in voice production, and two indicated only slightly improved voice production. As was seen in the original study, compliance played a large role in failure to improve, but the percentages of improved voices and decreased level of handicap were comparable in the two groups.

For the scientifically minded, the data for the original thirty-two subjects were statistically analyzed by a graduate student studying statistics at Texas A&M on May 29, 2010. He used the SAS system, paired TTEST procedure to examine the change in VHI scores pre- and post-clinic. The mean change was -34.65 points (p=<.000). An eighteen-point decrease is considered to be statistically significant. This analysis indicates a 95 percent confidence level that a person's perceived level of handicap will decrease with this program. The subject group was limited to those who did not select Botox or surgery as their preferred treatment following the clinic and included follow-up VHI scores for up to five years following the clinic.

As it currently stands, this method of treating SD is proving to be effective for the majority of people who use it. The improvements are not only significant but they stand up over the long term. There is variability in the length of time one needs to accomplish voice rehabilitation, and further studies are needed. In addition to the data collection and efficacy studies, I post personal testimonials on my website.

To stay up to date on these testimonials, visit my website at www.freetospeakvoicetherapy.com. I am in awe of some people who disappear after the clinic only to email or call me years later telling me how well their voices are coming along. There is no magic number of weeks, months, or years to voice rehabilitation. It is an ongoing management, but it puts the person with SD in control. Who with SD would not want to learn tools to increase control over his or her own voice? Botox treatment teaches dependence on a chemical and often results in a feeling of loss of control. I hear this from many of my patients, and the major reason they like voice rehabilitation is that they can see how the voice can be managed by their own strategies.

I attended my thirty-third high school reunion in 2009. One of my classmates told me she had seen my website and told a friend who had SD. Her friend purchased the book, studied it, applied the techniques, and recovered her voice. I was very happy to know this. I may never know how many people will find hope and healing through this method, but every story keeps me moving in the direction of my personal destiny. It is my responsibility to take what I have learned in my own life and share it.

Additionally, I talked to half my senior class that night and some of my high school teachers, and not one person commented on my voice. Most had no idea what I had gone through in 2004.

A few asked me how I got rid of my Alabama accent! That was easy compared to SD. It simply took about six months living in Minnesota and having to answer the question, "Where are you from?" on a daily basis! Perhaps that experience planted a seed in me that helped me realize the control that I had over my dialect that later would be directed toward my voice. Perhaps my attempts to change my accent started reorganizing my brain with regard to my voice. So many questions, so few answers!

Chapter 6
Case Studies in Voice Rehabilitation: Successes

For the purpose of confidentiality, case studies are presented without identifying information. Many of my clients are happy to provide personal references and their experiences of the clinic. For that information, please contact me via email at cpike200@gmail.com. All stories are entirely true. Ages are at the time of my initial evaluation/treatment. Statements in quotations are taken from the client's file or from personal correspondence. The following assessment information is expressed as the acronyms in bold, as follows, and is explained for those outside of the speech field:

1. Voice Handicap Index-30 (**VHI**). Developed and validated in 1997 by Barbara Jacobson and others, this is a self-rated instrument that analyzes a person's own perception of the level of handicap rendered by his or her voice dysfunction. Composed of three sections of ten questions each, it evaluates Function of the voice ("I use the phone less than I would like to"), Perceptual aspects of voice use ("I run out of air when I talk") and Emotional features ("I am tense talking to others because of my voice). The patient scores each item as 0=never, 1=almost never, 2=sometimes, 3=almost always, and 4=always. The total score indicates

that person's perceived level of handicap with regard to voice use. The range is 0 to 160. A score of less than 33 indicates no handicap. A change of 18 points is considered significant according to the developers of the test and, therefore, is used in our efficacy data.

2. Taylor-Johnson Psychosocial Assessment© (TJ), Psychological Publications, latest version 2007. This instrument can be taken online. The results are analyzed by our psychologist and discussed with the client. Psychological traits are presented based on self-response to a series of questions. There are nine separate areas, such as Nervous/Composed, Depressed/Light-Hearted, and Self-Disciplined/Impulsive. These give the counselor an idea of areas that could either contribute to success or interfere with it. A private consultation is offered each patient, and patients are given projects to help in specific areas of need.

Acoustic analysis was conducted using the **EZ Voice Plus** software© program from Voice Tek Enterprises, LLC, on a Dell Inspiron 710. A Samson R106 unidirectional microphone was positioned approximately two to three inches from the mouth. Fundamental frequency of connected speech (second sentence of the Rainbow passage), as well as jitter and shimmer for vowel (a 1.5-second clip of "ah") were used since normative data was provided based on these samples. Fundamental frequency is the average pitch of a person's voice. It may be higher or lower than the optimal pitch, which is determined during treatment. Jitter and shimmer are measured on the vowel "ah" and indicate variability in the pitch or loudness; they have some correlation with voice quality. For example, a high jitter measure is almost always present when a person has a vocal tremor. I present a variety of cases, beginning with the more successful ones and proceeding to cases where the program has not been sufficiently successful to date. Because it can take years for improvements to occur and because so many variables are involved in success rates, it may be best just to state the facts and let readers decide for themselves the possible "why" of success or failure. Since at this writing, I have seen more than 120 SD clients in either private consultation or in one of our clinics, it is hard to choose which to include. They are collectively valuable to me, and I have learned from each one. Regretfully, some never contact me after the clinic. Some disappear for years, and when I do hear from them, it can be good news or not. Some find it preferable or necessary to use Botox as their treatment of choice, and I do not see them as "failures." I fully support that method of treatment in some cases. For the purpose of success, and I consider myself in this group, the patient would have to describe a mostly normal voice and have a VHI score indicating no handicap (<33).

- **Case Study: Patient A**
  Patient A, male, age forty-four, was diagnosed with SD/ MTD by Donna Lundy, PhD, SLP at the University of Miami in January 2007. He had a history of spasmodic torticollis at age twenty-six, when he was finishing his PhD. It resolved after about a year without any active treatment. Seven years later, it returned as he was going through the tenure process. He had one Botox injection, and it resolved in about a year. A third bout of ST occurred seven years later and was more severe. Two Botox injections were unsuccessful, so he relied on biofeedback and physical therapy techniques developed by psychologist John Spencer. The neck condition slowly improved and at

the time of the clinic, he rated his neck recovery at around 80 to 90 percent.

Voice problems came on slowly at age forty-three, but a throat infection in late August 2006 exacerbated the problems. Initial ENT consultation found no physical problems. MRI of throat was negative. A second ENT specialist suggested acid reflux and prescribed Prevacid. Once he contacted Dr. Lundy, she recommended a trial of Botox. He received two small injections March 1 and March 29, 2007, and estimated the improvement to be around 10 percent. He also received voice therapy, which failed to help his condition. He then contacted me to schedule the intensive clinic and attended in July 2007.

A month prior to the clinic, he came in for evaluation and consultation and began to put the program into place. Post-onset of SD was approximately one year at the time of treatment. Subjective assessment of his conversational voice was that it was severely impaired and characteristic of adductor SD. As a lecturing professor, his voice was of utmost importance and had created situations during which he had been unable to lecture. VHI was 69 (Severe). TJ profile indicated high Anxiety and Depression scores (95th percentile) and low scores on Self-Discipline (15th percentile). Patient was highly motivated and believed in the holistic program. Acoustic analysis revealed fundamental frequency of 156 Hz (high), Jitter 1.9 (high), and Shimmer 1.4 (high).

Actual improvement during the clinic was judged to be around 25 percent, not a very big breakthrough. However, the patient left encouraged and ready to work at recovery. The psychologist met with him and gave him projects to help with the feelings of anxiety and depression. He also focused on strengthening his sense of identity, letting go of distractions, and pursuing passion in his life. Patient maintained contact with the breathing coach and the SLP via emails and voice clips.

Approximately six weeks following the clinic, with the school year approaching, the patient, in his own words, "panicked that I was not ready for teaching and decided to get a Botox shot. This was a mistake, as my voice is still not the same and it has been over four weeks. The shot has caused breathiness and weakness that persists. Where did I get this idea? Well, part of it is my own foolish impulsiveness, which can get me into trouble. Part of it was further reading of scientific journals that suggested the efficacy of combining Botox with voice therapy. So, that is where I headed but it was in the wrong direction. At least now I know that your approach is the only game in town, and I intend to follow it exclusively."

Luckily, the effects of the Botox diminished and he was able to resume his practice. He had been instructed to lower his pitch, breathe properly, participate in various activities to settle down his nervous system, and use resonant voicing. By January, his feedback indicated a decrease in VHI to 28 (no handicap) and significant improvement in the voice. One year after the clinic, the patient came in for a visit, and his voice quality was normal. I interviewed him and used his tapes to encourage others. VHI was 0 (perfect score). Acoustic analysis revealed fundamental frequency of 124 Hz, jitter .6, and shimmer .7, all well within the normal range. That was in July 2008 and, as of this writing, at age 47, his voice remains normal. He attributes his success to the holistic nature of the program, especially learning to be calm and slow down his nervous system. His neck condition is no longer an issue. Three years after the clinic, he continues to frequently email me about his continued success, stating that his voice is becoming even better than it was before SD.

- **Case Study: Patient B**

Patient B, female, age eighty-two, was diagnosed with spasmodic dysphonia by Dr. Herbert Dedo at UCMC in San Francisco in 2006. She reported a slow onset of voice difficulties beginning in 2004, worsening over time, but also variable. Her voice was hoarse, and she felt that it was jittery and hard to project. Dr. Izdebski, PhD, SLP conducted a voice evaluation, confirmed the diagnosis of adductor SD, and discussed voice therapy, Botox, and surgical procedures. She was told that voice therapy was very limited in helping with SD and she refused Botox because of its toxicity, so her last option was recurrent laryngeal nerve section, which was scheduled for July 18, 2006, at UCSF/Mt. Zion Medical Center.

Meanwhile, the patient's adult children began researching options and found out about our clinic online. They told her they did not want her to have surgery but, rather, to attend a clinic. She reviewed the information and enthusiastically enrolled in the January 2007 clinic, canceling the surgery. Subjectively, her voice was strained with a significant intermittent tremor. She was a retired teacher, twice divorced and now single, in excellent health and very active. Her TJ was completely normal with regard to her psychosocial profile. Of significance, she was extremely composed and self-disciplined. VHI was 59 (high moderate).

Acoustic analysis revealed fundamental frequency of 177 Hz (low), jitter .73 (slightly high), and shimmer .88 (high). She was instructed to elevate her pitch, use resonant voice techniques, and breathe appropriately, voicing without tensing her abdominal muscles. We also discussed the possibility of unrealized past trauma, and she remembered that the voice problems started when her son-in-law was killed in a hit-and-run accident while biking, followed by the deaths of several other loved ones. She had also taken a hard fall around that time, which frightened her.

By the end of five days, she felt her voice had improved 95 percent. Her tremor decreased significantly when she learned to relax her entire body when speaking. At six months, her VHI was 32 (no handicap), and almost four years later, at age 85, she continues to be pleased with her results from the clinic. A recent email stated, "I am so proud that you started me on my way to improving the SD which was bothering me immensely before I attended your class. I go merrily on my way now, singing to start the day. Talking with friends and strangers is much, much easier and I take command, not feeling that I will have a problem speaking."

- **Case Study: Patient C**

Patient C, male, age fifty-eight, had a history of voice problems beginning in July 2005, at age fifty-six, which started as hoarseness and the perceived need to clear his throat. The first six months, several medical doctors told him that he had allergies. An ENT consultant diagnosed throat infection and allergies. An initial videostroboscopy was normal. In May 2006, he saw an ENT at the Mayo Clinic in Scottsdale who also said that allergies were the culprit. He also recommended voice therapy, but the patient was traveling and unable to schedule it at the time. While researching voice problems online, the patient came across information about SD. It was getting very difficult to talk and he was feeling strangled, so he asked the ENT about it. It was suggested that he might have SD, although mild, and he began some voice therapy. He purchased my book and his voice therapist worked with him using the techniques, as well as contacting me to see if I felt he would benefit from the intensive clinic. Meanwhile, he had a consultation with another speech therapist, who told him Botox was the gold standard of treatment and that voice therapy was not a successful treatment for SD.

Patient C attended the clinic in May 2007. His TJ was insignificant, but high in Inhibition. VHI was 71 (severe). He was able to identify some stressors leading up to his voice problems, such as retirement, extensive travel in an RV, and the deaths of his in-laws. He noted that when he felt nervous, his voice would worsen. Subjectively, his voice quality was strained with some noticeable breaks. Fundamental frequency was 156 Hz (high), jitter 2.1 (high), and shimmer 2.0 (high). Within a few days of being instructed to speak in a lower pitch with attention to improve breath support (inhibit the tendency to gasp and heave), resonate without forcing, and let go of anticipatory anxiety, the patient was conversing normally. He was able to lower his pitch to 112 Hz (normal) and decrease jitter to .73 (slightly high), and shimmer by 50 percent. Voice breaks were virtually eliminated by the end of the clinic. The patient was pleased and encouraged.

However, soon after the clinic, the patient's only child, who had just given birth to his first grandchild, was diagnosed with lupus. He and his wife were called on to help her and the baby. He was very stressed and worried over her condition and had no time or desire to work on his voice. At the six-month follow-up, he was not doing well. His voice had become difficult again. I encouraged him to recognize how this emotional jolt was affecting his progress and to try to let go of the worry and take time for his voice rehabilitation. One year after the clinic, a completely different picture emerged. He stated, "My voice is doing much better and has been serving me well. What helps me best is to let go and not get stressed every time I want to speak. I just go for it and it works well most of the time. I think of my experience at the clinic every day and I thank you and Mike for all your help and encouragement."

At that time, his VHI was 27 (no handicap), and he rated his voice as significantly improved. He had, however, begun to have some problems breathing and which sounded like it could be paradoxical vocal fold movement disorder. He described that he felt as if his vocal folds were closing up when he was inhaling. He had been evaluated, and the doctor found nothing wrong. A recent email stated, "My voice has been fine for over a year now, but I still have problems with the breathing."

- **Case Study: Patient D**
Patient D, female, fifty-seven, reported a sudden onset following laryngitis in February 2005. She denied any stressors other than her voice affecting her work and social life. She was officially diagnosed with SD in May 2005 by Dr. Gregg Govett. This diagnosis was confirmed by

another ENT who specializes in SD. She had some short-term voice therapy that did not help. Her diagnosis was abductor SD, and her voice was weak and low in pitch with breathy voice breaks. Severity was moderate, as she had periods of normal voicing. She attended the first clinic held in August 2005. VHI was 60 (high moderate), fundamental frequency was 189 (slightly low) and range was extremely limited, jitter 1.28 (high), and shimmer .22 (normal).

She was instructed to elevate her pitch to 200 Hz or higher, use more inflection, stop pushing through the breaks, coordinate the breath with the voice, and practice glides to increase her range. The first clinic was only three and a half days, yet she felt her voice free up and rated it at 70 percent improved by the end of the sessions. She continued to slowly and steadily progress, practicing daily, which included singing exercises. At six months, her VHI was 1 (no handicap), and she rated her voice as normal. More than four years later, she reports that her voice continues to function normally. A recent email stated, "I think of you and the group quite often; your seminar was a life-changing event for me. My voice is at 95 percent or better, every now and then, when I am tired or on the phone, I mess up. I just pull up my courage, pitch my voice, and try again. I cannot thank you enough for what you did for me. When I attended your clinic, I wanted to be able to read to my grandchildren. I can, and they love it." As of October 2009, she rated her voice as normal, and she is no longer doing any type of exercise. She reports only occasional struggles with the voice when under stress or illness but can easily "gather myself and start over and my voice is fine."

- **Case Study: Patient E**

  Patient E, a female PE coach, age thirty-six, had a gradual deterioration of voice beginning in April 2006. Initially she was told she had allergies then voice overuse and, after a year of continuing difficulties and a voice that was cutting in and out, Dr. Patty Lee diagnosed her with adductor SD. She recommended Botox injections, which the patient declined. She attended the clinic in July 2007. Her TJ was unremarkable, but she described herself as a perfectionist. Her voice problems were very upsetting to her and she was almost unable to teach. She was becoming short of breath and anxious about speaking. VHI was 82 (severe), fundamental frequency was 152 Hz (low), jitter was 1.16 (high), and shimmer was 1.21 (high). She had very shallow, tight, reversed breathing patterns and was trying to push out her voice.

  She was instructed to elevate her pitch to the level of her normal hum, which was around 190 Hz, release tensions, and use proper breathing techniques. Stressors around the time of onset were discussed. As she recognized the emotional connection to breathing and voice as well as the mechanics she needed, she was able to quickly make adjustments so that by the end of the clinic, acoustics had changed significantly with fundamental frequency of 186 Hz (low normal), jitter .9 (slightly high) and shimmer decreased slightly. At six months, VHI had decreased to 32, and she rated her voice as significantly improved. I had the opportunity to see her again two years after the clinic. She was maintaining a fundamental frequency of 186 Hz with normal jitter and shimmer measures, and her voice had no abnormal qualities. VHI had further decreased to

21. She reported that she felt her voice was significantly improved to normal. She stated, "When my voice needs an adjustment, I use the techniques I learned at the clinic. It's not consistent because I only do it when needed. Just a little tweaking with breathing and I get back on track with my voice."

• **Case Study: Patient F**

Patient F, male, a pastor aged fifty-three, had a lengthy history of voice difficulties dating back to 1993, when he was forty years old. Initial consultations with various ENT doctors resulted in diagnosis of acid reflux and subsequent medications. Videostroboscopy was suggestive of vocal fold bowing and slight atrophy. Voice therapy was recommended. He saw two different speech therapists for several months each with no improvement. One doctor suggested medialization surgery, which the patient refused. Dr. Peak Woo, at Mt. Sinai Hospital in New York, was consulted in October 2004 and diagnosed the patient with adductor SD. He was told that voice therapy would not help and that his normal voice would never return. Botox was recommended, but the patient declined.

This patient tried alternative methods such as chiropractic, nutritional, and massage therapies to no avail. In February 2005, he spent two weeks with Morton Cooper, PhD, SLP, and reported moderate improvement, but it was mostly temporary. Dr. Cooper suggested that he return, so he spent an additional two weeks with him in August 2005. Only slight improvements were reported during the second session. He was forced to stop preaching in October 2005. In March 2006, he began working with a singing teacher, Alma Vejas, who had recovered from SD herself. She used the Smolover method with him for four months. His voice returned, but he continued to feel effort in voicing and breathing. He attended our clinic in October 2006. Voice quality was subjectively good at the assessment. His TJ was unremarkable. VHI was 59 (moderate). Acoustic analysis revealed fundamental frequency of 122 Hz (normal), jitter 1.09 (high), and shimmer .27 (normal). Patient described a feeling of effort in voicing, and frequent but brief hesitations were noted. He had returned to preaching but felt that he was unable to "get my breath to support and work with my voice." He had a very tight diaphragm and shallow breathing. His larynx had a tendency to elevate frequently as he spoke, which probably contributed to the hesitations. He was instructed to lower his pitch to keep the larynx low, visualizing a low larynx, continue with his singing instruction, and follow Mike's breathing protocols. At the end of the clinic, he maintained a fundamental frequency of 110 Hz (normal) with slight decreases in jitter and shimmer.

Over the next several years, the patient would call or send periodic emails, updating me on his progress. We discussed problems as they occurred and would troubleshoot. He did the same with Mike, as he felt that his breathing had needed the most attention when he attended our clinic. He continued diligent practice and preaching/teaching and, eight months after the clinic, VHI had decreased to 6. Problems were strictly perceptual, and no one noted any problems with his voice. To date, his voice is fully functional. VHI in October 2009 was 7 (no handicap), and he rated it as normal despite very high voice use on a daily basis. I enjoy his Sunday morning phone calls when I am having a clinic, as he encourages me and assures me that his success has been maintained.

• **Case Study: Patient G**

Patient G, female, age fifty-one, working full-time as a vice president of nursing, described a gradual voice deterioration beginning in 2001. Her physician felt it was anxiety-related and prescribed an antidepressant. An allergist suggested decongestants, and her initial fiberoptic laryngoscopy was unremarkable. She saw a speech therapist who suggested that her vocal cords were dry and provided some short-term therapy. None of these helped her voice and, in January of 2006, she was finally diagnosed with adductor SD with tremor by Dr. Keith Wilson. She started treatment with Botox the next month and received injections in February, May, July, and October 2006. She had just scheduled a fifth injection when she found information about our clinic on the internet. Because she was frustrated by the side effects of the injections (no voice for up to six weeks) and inconsistent improvement, she attended the clinic in January 2007. When she called and left a message on my voicemail, her voice was subjectively tight and tremulous with voice breaks. It had been three months since her last injection.

Patient G had a VHI of 100 (severe). She described years of using strategies to try to improve her voice such as elevating her pitch and using a singsong voice or short phrases. She would also tell people she was sick if they inquired about her hoarseness. She felt she was "crazy" or imagining the problems until she received the proper diagnosis. Her TJ profile was high in Anxiety (90th percentile) and in Inhibition. When she arrived for the initial evaluation, her voice quality was a bit tremulous but did not sound particularly strained. She stated that as she went to pick up her rental car, her voice came out loud and clear; she had a feeling that she was here to recover her voice and that recovery had already begun.

Acoustic analysis revealed fundamental frequency of 225 Hz (normal), jitter 1.29 (high), and shimmer .85 (high). Focus and resonance were fairly good. She had considerable problems coordinating her breathing with her voice. Much of the voice therapy sessions were spent discussing how stressors had contributed to her voice problems and that some of the compensations she had been using were actually helping her re-groove the voice. She had a lot of anticipatory anxiety at work regarding her voice and felt she was faking and trying to hide her problem. What she was actually doing was using her voice in a different manner than what felt automatic or natural to her. The higher pitch and singsong voice masked the symptoms she felt. The others in her group were impressed with the quality of her voice as she tried to convince us she really did have SD! When her sister called her on her cellular phone, we all stood in awe of the immediate deterioration of her voice. We heard a smooth clear voice quickly become shaky and strangled, and it was a lesson to us all how situational SD could be. Triggers such as certain people or situations in our lives could affect the voice. Patient G left confident that she had mastered the techniques she needed to control her voice. Seven months after the clinic, her VHI had decreased 69 points and was then 31. She considered her voice moderately improved (80 percent) at that point and had been without a Botox injection for eleven months. She stated that her ENT was captivated by the improvement she had attained. Two years after the clinic, she stated, "My voice is not perfect, but 90 percent improved since a couple of years ago before my Botox adventure. I am able to do public speaking in an auditorium. I can look back and understand my issues were largely stress related. I still utilize the techniques learned. Sometimes I simply need to stop and relax and use my diaphragm properly for breathing."

- **Case Study: Patient H**

  Patient H, female, age thirty-nine, had an onset of voice difficulties dating back to 2001 at the age of thirty-one. The year before, when she was eight months pregnant, the father of her child left her. She had a business in one city but moved to another and subsequently had a crisis (new city, lost control of business, single mother). Her voice began to change, and she described it as shaky and sounding as if she were going to cry, even if she did not feel upset. Voice problems continued to wax and wane, often depending on emotional states. She saw a speech therapist who was unable to help her and believed that her problem was largely emotional.

  By 2006, she was very frustrated and stated in her case history, "I started looking on the internet and found Dr. Morton Cooper. I booked myself to go to California and stayed a month in 2006. I recovered about 50 percent of my voice by the time I left. However, he did not give me ' a step-by-step program to continue and when I got back, stress took over and my voice took a back seat. I did try to keep up the basic exercises I learned from Dr. Cooper, but could not continue for more than a few weeks. My voice continued to vary day to day, with my telephone voice terrible. I've started and restarted the Cooper exercises so many times until I lost all motivation to do them."

Patient H had not tried Botox when she attended the voice intensive in June 2008. She was taking Rivotril for restless leg syndrome and was having weekly massage therapy. Her VHI was 63 (severe). Her TJ profile indicated slightly high in Depression (60th percentile), as well as high Impulsivity and Indifference. Acoustic analysis indicated fundamental frequency of 164 Hz (low), jitter 1.08 (high), and shimmer 1.2 (high). Her stomach and diaphragm were noted to be extremely tense while voicing. Breath support was poor. She reported that speaking was extremely effortful.

Our breathing coach instructed Patient H in how to breathe and coordinate breath and the voice effectively. She was instructed in using a higher pitch and the singsong intonation she had discovered, staying calm when speaking, and understanding the connection between her emotional state and her voice. Strategies were discussed because it was clear that her lack of self-discipline prevented her from practice. She experienced normal voicing with the therapists and the group during the clinic.

The patient provided feedback eight months after the clinic, at which time her VHI had decreased by 48 points to a score of 15. She reported that her voice was significantly better and that friends and family judged it as normal. In long-term follow up in May 2009, almost one year later, she stated, "I am happy to give you feedback that I still have a fully functional voice, something I rarely think of. The odd time it goes a bit croaky, I find myself noticing it, and it helps to relax, unwind the tension because it usually happens in a stressful situation, and listen to what the other person is saying rather than jumping in, reacting, and trying desperately to get myself heard. No one I know or meet would know that I have SD, which is awesome."

- **Case Study: Patient I**

Patient I, female, age forty-seven, had been diagnosed with abductor SD by Dr. Sanford Archer. She described problems since April 2006, when she would lose sounds in her middle range. In February 2007, ten months later, she had an upper respiratory infection with laryngitis and her voice worsened. She then saw both her general doctor and an ENT, who suspected SD but first sent her to a speech therapist. After two months of therapy, she was referred to Dr. Archer, who prescribed a steroid and antihistamine. Her general doctor prescribed medication for reflux. None of the medications helped, and she felt that her voice was worsening. She was working full-time as an environmental biologist and was running a farm. When she returned to Dr. Archer, he diagnosed her in February 2007 and explained that Botox was the treatment of choice. She declined and looked for other options. She found the clinic via the internet and attended in November 2007.

She presented with a VHI of 113 (very high). Acoustic analysis revealed fundamental frequency of 166 Hz (low), jitter 1.6 (high), and shimmer 1.6 (high). She was unable to sustain a vowel for more than a second before becoming aphonic. Her voice had many breathy breaks, and she struggled to speak. Her TJ profile was high in Anxiety (92nd percentile) and Inhibition. While her Depression score was unremarkable, her affect was one of sadness, and her posture slumped inward. Breathing was shallow with a very tight solar plexus. She stated that her husband of 21 years died suddenly of a massive heart attack in December 2005 and about four months later her voice became affected. She had not been sleeping well and was worrying a lot about the farm and her ability to work without an adequate voice. She did not feel that her voice problems were related to emotions around her husband's death, although she was commonly asked this question. However, she felt that not having a voice was greatly affecting her self-esteem, social life, and ability to do her job.

The patient was not taking medications but was visiting a chiropractor, who was working with her shoulders and back. She felt that her voice was better after the treatments. She admitted at the clinic that she was often overwhelmed by grief and subsequent emotions and had not had any grief counseling.

The breathing coach found that she needed a lot of work in balancing her breathing and that it would help with the anxiety. She was instructed to elevate her pitch, and to work through hums, trills, and engaging the vocal folds. She worked on releasing bodily tensions and coordinating the breath with the voice, doing so without pushing. She was instructed to take it slow in her practice with voiceless consonants and practice at the single word level until she was very comfortable. The psychologist suggested grief counseling and possibly medication for anxiety.

The patient was very compliant and truly put together a holistic program with our guidance. She improved her diet, sleep, and physical fitness, and began to get regular massage therapy and to participate in yoga. She used a mild anti-anxiety medication as needed. She practiced positive affirmations, breathing, and voice exercises, and experienced steady improvement. A month after the clinic, she felt her voice was at about 50 percent, and others began to comment on both her voice and her physical appearance improving. By six months, her VHI had decreased 105 points and was only an 8. She felt that by that time, her voice was normal 90 percent of the time and was significantly better at its worst.

As of this writing, she continues to have a fully functioning voice, perceptually normal to others and very rarely a problem. She feels she is back to being herself now, with ample social engagements, working, and even singing in a choir. With each success, there is hope.

Chapter 7
Case Studies: Partial Successes (On the Path)

These studies represent clients who reported benefit from the program. Most of them made significant progress with voice production. Many still feel considerably handicapped with regard to their voices, and some are currently using Botox treatments to help manage their condition. Some consider themselves still on the road to recovery since they have been working with the program for a year or less.

- **Case History: Patient J**
  Patient J, a female attorney aged forty-nine, with MTD/SD diagnosis, was referred by her speech-language pathologist. With onset of symptoms in 2003, it took her quite a long time to get a diagnosis. She had a history of very high voice use in demanding situations with her profession, coupled with many social and volunteer events. Giving her voice problem the proper "title" appeared to be a subject of great debate, and she had taken several Botox injections, which helped temporarily. She was in voice therapy. She attended the clinic in June 2006. Her voice was subjectively very strained and with many voice breaks. She spoke with great effort. Acoustic analysis revealed a fundamental frequency 243 Hz (high average), jitter 1.5 (high), and shimmer .45

(high). Breathing was very restricted. The patient was highly motivated to succeed. VHI was 67 (severe), and her TJ was unremarkable. She was instructed in coordinating the voice with breath and allowing easy airflow both with and without voice. She was told to use more intonation in her voice and trained in confidential voice and resonant voice techniques. She was very successful during the clinic; her voice improved 70 percent and she was very pleased and encouraged that she could re-groove her voice by using the rehabilitation techniques she had learned. She did exceptionally well with the confidential voice techniques, which virtually eliminated voice breaks.

After the clinic, she was diligent in her practice and took a leave from work. She continued in voice-demanding roles, however, and found it very difficult to give them up. She would practice, then spend hours each day speaking with the SD voice. She had difficulty in carrying over into conversation the level of quality of her practice. At the initial follow-up, she had demonstrated some improvement, which varied from day to day. She continued to follow up over time and, by six to eight months, she was at about 75 percent of where she wished to be with her voice.

Returning to her job really set her back. By January 2008, her VHI was 56 (moderate), her fundamental frequency had decreased to 191 Hz (slightly low), jitter was 1.9 (high), and shimmer was 1.3 (high). She decided to return to the clinic in February 2008 for a refresher course to get back on track. She felt she benefited from the breathing and voice instruction as well as being with others who were experiencing SD. She left determined to make the program work for her. Despite her best efforts, she was unable to gain the control she needed to meet her voice demands.

She decided to try Botox again. She received a dose of 2.5 u unilaterally. She experienced breathy voice followed by a period of improvement around thirteen weeks. She sent me an audio sample, and it was definitely the best I had heard her voice since the end of the first clinic. She continues with regular Botox injections and is also continuing voice rehabilitation exercises. She is pleased but hopes to be able to discontinue the injections eventually. A recent summary from this patient tells it from her perspective.

"As of February 2009, it has now been almost 5 years since my diagnosis of AD/SD. Although the ENT who specialized in voice suggested speech therapy prior to the only other option of Botox, his default position was clearly a Botox injection. Although I tried speech therapy first, in hindsight, the time suggested for voice exercises yet without suggested change in amount of daily voice use simply could not work. I had extremely intensive voice demands of my profession (namely, a prosecuting attorney) and in my extra-curricular activities. I eventually tried 3 Botox injections but with minimal and very short-term benefits.

It was suggested that I try more intensive voice therapy that led me to a very progressive speech/language pathologist who discovered Connie Pike's clinic and recommended I give it a try. By this time, I had gone through 2 years of entrenching voice behaviors that attempted to compensate for my SD but, in fact, worsened my condition. Nevertheless, after two visits to the clinic and a personal session, improvement was made. Although efforts were made to adjust voice use, including taking a leave from work, by the time I made the necessary adjustments to my voice, I was back at work. I felt that positive changes had been made although I was not able to converse easily at work. In October 2008, I tried Botox again and was able to communicate more easily.

I am convinced that the 2 years of voice work following Connie's program contributed to the benefits I now experience with Botox. Botox is by no means a cure nor has it brought back my original voice entirely. The voice is weak and breathy for 2 weeks and it not always consistent, nor do I have the singing voice that I miss terribly. But I remember the tools Connie gave me and I try to use them on a daily basis to entrench those positive breathing and voicing techniques during the duration of the Botox. The ENT and speech pathologist appear to be extremely pleased with my results and I am thrilled with the ability to communicate again.

I regret that I was not able to overcome this without the use of Botox. I suppose the biggest regret is not having learned about Connie's clinic at the outset of my diagnosis. I firmly believe I would have been able to achieve the kind of success she has, but that is in the past and I need to look forward."

- **Case Study: Patient K**

  Patient K, female, age fifty-six, has an extremely complex psychosocial and medical history. She had problems with her family of origin (her mother had repeated nervous breakdowns, and she was forced to share a bedroom with her parents until age fourteen). She had been married three times, had been a single mother of two boys for a time, had recently remarried, and was caring for an elderly father and grandmother as well. Her history of stated significant stressors spanned decades. She worked full-time as a manager of a mortgage company and, a self-described workaholic, had a history of yearly URIs when she would lose her voice for two to four weeks, yet continue to work, whispering if she had to.

Voice problems became more consistent in fall 2006. Prior medical history was significant for insomnia, high cholesterol, pre-diabetes, and essential tremors in her legs (restless leg syndrome). She was diagnosed with SD at the Vanderbilt Clinic in January 2007. The speech therapist there told her that no amount of voice therapy would help her and suggested Botox as the only viable treatment. She was taking several medications for her conditions. She initially refused Botox treatment for the SD, tried gabapentin (600 mg), and had extensive psychological counseling for family of origin and divorce issues. She attended the clinic in August 2008.

The patient reported chronic fatigue and the desire to lose weight. Her voice dysfunction was significantly handicapping. Her VHI score was 113. Her TJ indicated high Anxiety, Inhibition, and Hostility. Self-discipline was high and depression low. Acoustic analysis revealed fundamental frequency of 195 Hz (slightly low), jitter 1.2 (high), and shimmer .54 (high). She described moderate to severe effort in vocalizing. Stress seemed to be a common theme in our sessions together, and we discussed how she might decrease this. Subjective assessment of the voice indicated tense, effortful voice production with shallow breathing but no voice breaks.

She was instructed to lift and lighten her pitch to around 220 Hz. She learned how to breathe properly and to release the breath, as well as varied strategies to help her feel calmer overall (activating the parasympathetic nervous system). In the clinic environment, she felt safe and free, and her voice improved dramatically. She was able to converse with her fellow participants easily 90 percent of the time by the last day. She agreed to take a month off work, feeling that her voice had improved 80 percent overall; she wanted to make sure she maintained those gains.

Her early emails indicated success. Unfortunately, life took over as she returned to her demanding job. She continued to have challenges over the next year. Physically, she had recurrent upper respiratory infections, an abnormal mammogram, and allergies. She reported feeling pressured by medical personnel at Vanderbilt to have Botox shots for her voice, but participated in a sleep study that revealed a mild case of sleep apnea. She was then counseled against Botox, with warnings that she could strangle in the night when an episode of apnea occurred if she had used it. At the eight-month follow-up, her VHI had decreased by 34 points yet remained in the severe range at 79. She reported being 50 percent compliant to her program yet too caught up in her busy life. She continued to desire to control her voice herself and, in October 2009, stated, "I am actually getting my voice back again, and with a lot of hard work, I am going to beat this thing called SD and without Botox." She rated her voice as moderately improved, anywhere from 60 to 80 percent and stated, "I just have to remember to take care of myself and all I have learned, keep it simple, eat well, and sleep well. When I do this, I am speaking more like my old self. People comment on how much better I sound, which gives me hope."

At only a little over a year, it was too soon to tell if voice rehabilitation would be a success, and there were numerous variables in her complex case. She quickly attained an almost normal or normal voice production in the safe cocoon of the clinic, yet found it very difficult to carry over into her busy life. Currently, she continues to get periodic evaluations at Vanderbilt and her current diagnosis is vocal tremor with mild SD. She is participating in Qigong and painting lessons to help her relax and has lost weight. She reports communicating well in face to face situations, but that the heavy telephone use that her job requires is an enemy. She continues to feel handicapped by the inconsistency in her voice but is not considering Botox treatments. She continues to use the breathing and voice exercises she learned at the clinic and is beginning to take Inderal for the tremors in her legs and voice.

- **Case Study: Patient L**
  Patient L, a female accountant aged thirty-nine, reported voice difficulties that began during a divorce fifteen years before she was diagnosed. She stated that during that time, she had problems expressing her emotions. Once the divorce was resolved, her voice improved. She noticed some problems with public speaking, and the voice deteriorated during another period of stress in 2005 when she was thirty-seven, which is when she was diagnosed with AD/SD. By this time, she had remarried and had two elementary-age children. She had about five speech therapy sessions, which did not help. She had two Botox injections in 2007 and also tried alternative therapies such as acupuncture, Reike, massage, and chiropractic treatments. Only Botox helped her voice production. She was taking no medications.

The patient was interested in our holistic program and attended the August 2008 clinic. In a pre-clinic questionnaire, she expressed concern that her fear of speaking and being judged, lack of self-confidence, and shyness might prevent her from being successful with the program. She presented with a VHI of 91 (severe), and her TJ indicated high Anxiety (71st percentile) and Depression (67th percentile), and significant Inhibition, Submissiveness, and Impulsivity. Subjectively, her voice was tensely focused in the throat and low in pitch. Fundamental frequency was 188 Hz (low), jitter .79 (high), and shimmer .72 (high). She was instructed to elevate her pitch, restructure her breathing patterns, and recognize the emotional component to her voice difficulties. She was successful with both confidential voice and resonant voice, focusing her voice up out of her throat.

At follow-up, she reported moderate improvement and more control. She had not, however, viewed her DVD from the clinic "because I did not want to see it," and she did not take advantage of the follow-up, although she felt she needed ongoing regular support after the clinic to succeed. She reported 50 percent compliance to the prescribed program. Frustrated by her continued difficulty in talking, she decided to get a Botox shot in January 2009: "because I needed a break from SD." She lost her voice for ten days, after which she had three months of a "perfect voice." As she began to struggle, she used the voice and breathing techniques she learned at the clinic and began to notice that her voice was good when she was relaxed and bad when she was rushing about or nervous and stressed. Six months after the injection, she felt that all the effects had worn off, and she had more control over her voice than before, but not consistently. She has not decided whether she will return for more Botox treatment. This patient is an excellent example of the two treatments working well together. What was recommended and what may be missing is some psychological counseling and possible medication to address the anxiety, depression, and other emotional factors contributing to the patient's overall health.

- **Case Study: Patient M**

Patient M, a male chaplain aged sixty, had experienced voice difficulties since 1992. Despite participating in speech therapy for several years, his voice continued to deteriorate, and the speech therapist suggested he might have spasmodic dysphonia. A clinical psychologist also evaluated the patient but found no psychological reason for the voice difficulties. The patient's wife saw an article on laryngeal dystonia in the newspaper, leading him to consult with several otolaryngologists where he lived in Scotland. In September 1995, he was diagnosed with adductor laryngeal dystonia and began botulinum toxin treatments (Dysport) in October 1995. He had "miraculous" improvements in his voice as a result of the first injection but less reliable results for subsequent injections. The National Healthcare System only approved injections once every six months, so the patient had to manage on his own much of the time and retired from the Church of Scotland in 1998. His last injection in May 2007 gave him little relief. He attended the clinic in late July 2007 after hearing me speak at a dystonia meeting in London.

The patient presented with a VHI of 63 (severe), and his TJ was unremarkable. Acoustic analysis revealed fundamental frequency of 134 Hz (normal), jitter 2.5 (high), and shimmer 1.2 (high). His temperament was gregarious, and he was quite confident that he could control his voice without continuing with the injections. He experimented with a lower pitch and resonant voice techniques. Trills were used to loosen overly tight articulators. Breathing techniques addressed overly tight abdominals and lack of full, deep breathing. Singing exercises appeared to help him considerably.

He was quite pleased with the gains he made at the clinic and reported that people noticed the improvements in his voice right away, including his ENT consultant when he visited in August and canceled upcoming injections. He was speaking effortlessly for the first three or four months but began to encounter some mild difficulties after that time. We discussed that he may have been still experiencing some effects from the May injection when he attended the clinic in July, even though he did not perceive it. By November, when he would have received another injection, he was beginning to feel slight catches on some words. He stated that before voice rehabilitation, these would have been full spasms. He was diligent in keeping us informed of problems so we could troubleshoot with him. The patient had been serving as the Scotland Manager of The Dystonia Society in the UK, and he advocated voice rehabilitation. He was impressed with research being conducted in the UK suggesting holistic or alternative treatments for other focal dystonias.

Follow-up VHI had decreased to 30 (no handicap). Gains were maintained and, in August 2009, he stated, "I have not had Botox since attending the clinic and I don't worry about my voice quality now. Having said that, I am constantly working at producing a spasm-free voice. I attend to posture, breathing, throat configuration, and taking the voice to the front of the mouth. It is worse in the morning, but by the time I am in public, most people are unaware that there is a problem. I would say that my voice is improved about 85 percent. Although I am working to produce good voice, I am not physically exhausted by doing so as was the case before."

I recently asked the patient whether he placed himself in the successful or partially successful category due to the inconsistency and effort he was experiencing. He had met his goal of eliminating the Botox treatments, and his VHI indicated there was no longer a handicap. However, he described periods of difficulty producing voice and stated, "I would agree with your assessment that I would be in the partially successful category. I had a very good spring and summer where people who did not know I had a problem would not have noticed. About four weeks ago, quite suddenly, my symptoms returned with a vengeance and I have been struggling to speak. Looking back, I have had something similar at about the same time of year for the past several years. As autumn approaches and the temperature falls, I have a dystonic spasm in my abdomen, which affects my breath control. It is improving a bit and I hope to get back to my previous post-clinic state soon."

The patient stated that he could still sing well and talk loudly without a problem but struggled in moderating his volume in conversation.

- **Case Study: Patient N**

  Patient N, female, forty-two, was diagnosed with adductor SD at the University of Washington approximately two and a half years before attending the clinic in February 2008. The year before diagnosis, she had problems with vocal tremor. In 2005, she had a severe episode of obsessive compulsive disorder. She had one Botox injection but found it very painful, so she had begun to explore alternatives. She had been receiving acupuncture treatments and medications to help with anxiety and depression (Buspar and Pamelor). She had been under stress with her job in a dental front office and described a strong relationship between her level of stress and her voice.

  The patient presented with a VHI of 86 (severe). TJ indicated high Anxiety (83rd percentile), Depression (82nd percentile), Inhibition, and Submissiveness. Her breathing was shallow and restricted by a tight diaphragm and abdominal muscles. She tended to try to push out her voice by tensing her stomach. Acoustic analysis revealed fundamental frequency 191 Hz (low), jitter 1.6 (high), and shimmer 1.8 (high). When she pitched her voice to the level of her hum, it was 247 Hz, so she was instructed to elevate her pitch, improve resonance, sweep up and down scales, and release identified tensions. The breathing coach found many areas that needed work. The relationship between her emotional state and her voice was discussed, and she was given reading material on reframing negative thought patterns and using affirmations. Anticipatory anxiety in speaking situations was also affecting her. She found an effortless hum and was able to use hum/speaking techniques.

The patient's initial feedback at eight months indicated that she felt that her voice was moderately improved. Her VHI had not significantly decreased as expected. She stated that she had a hard time completing it because of the variability of her voice day to day: "Some days I have a pretty normal voice day and other days it feels like I've taken 10 steps backward." She had been fairly compliant in her voice exercises for the first month or two after the clinic but had tapered off quickly after that time. An email nineteen months after the clinic stated, "Since attending the clinic, I have definitely made progress. Some days are better than others. Yet remembering your advice that 'a bad voice day does not a bad voice make' helps. I have also made progress in talking in groups of people. That has come with MUCH effort, but with perseverance, relaxing/breathing as I talk, and prayer, I am happy to say that it is getting easier. I definitely am glad I attended your clinic and believe it gave me the determination to not let SD own me."

- **Case Study: Patient O**
  Patient O, a female full-time Christian Science practitioner aged fifty-three, reported voice difficulties dating back to 2001, when she was forty-seven years old. She was teaching third grade and had progressive difficulty speaking until she was completely aphonic and had to write to communicate. She saw an ENT in 2003, who referred her for speech therapy. She tried it for a while, but her voice did not improve. All along, she was having prayer-based Christian Science treatment. She described short periods of normal voicing alternating with periods of time when "it is like a wall rises up in my throat and I can't get past it

without straining, and that makes my throat sore and my head ache."

The patient had divorced an abusive husband and had three adult children. She was living with her mother at the time of the clinic but described her life as relatively stress-free despite many prior years of extreme stress. She had been forced to change careers due to her voice failing. She enrolled in the clinic in May 2007, hoping to be able to learn techniques to better control her voice. She presented with a VHI of 69 (severe). Her TJ profile was relatively unremarkable. She appeared composed and self-disciplined but scored fairly high in Inhibition.

Subjectively, the patient was hardly able to produce sound. Her cadence was slow and speech halting as she struggled to produce voice. Her entire body was very tense, and her breathing was shallow. Acoustic analysis revealed fundamental frequency of 184 Hz (low), jitter 1.9 (high), and shimmer .86 (high). She realized the need to open to the possibility of receiving help. She did well with humming and resonant voice techniques, using "m" words for resonance and "h" to increase airflow. She was instructed to elevate her pitch to target 200 Hz and to practice hum/ speak techniques. She had some breakthrough experiences with the breathing coaching and singing. She left with a connected fundamental frequency of 203 Hz (normal) and more of a flow to her speech.

This patient did not provide feedback upon request. She did not respond to the group emails, and I did not hear from her until almost two years after the clinic. In an email, she apologized, "for being one of the disappearing clients" and stated that her voice was closely tied to the amount of stress she was experiencing. She said that, presently, "the wall that blocked my voice and breathing is always down," and that she was using her voice more and it kept getting stronger. She said she had learned valuable tools at the clinic to understand how her voice and breathing should behave, so she could learn to monitor them and make adjustments.

The patient became more comfortable sharing her successes over the next six months and currently reports that she is "constantly getting comments about how much better my voice is now." She sent an audio file for me to review, and the change was subjectively much better. She reported that she had finally decided that she could talk and that her perception of her own voice was often worse than how it sounded to others. Overall, she was speaking well and participating in board meetings and easy conversations with friends. She had most difficulty projecting her voice without it becoming "scratchy." She reported that although her voice was not perfect, it was 100 percent functional. However, she would like to improve her tone and pitch.

In late October 2009, almost two and a half years after the clinic, she returned the feedback. She rated her voice as significantly improved, and her VHI had decreased 34 points to 35 (mild). She stated, "Success may not be what you think it is. The voice is there. Getting to it and setting it free might not be the same thing, but both are possible!"

- **Case Study: Patient P**
  Patient P, female, thirty-eight, began to have symptoms of voice dysfunction in October 2005. It took her about nine months to get a diagnosis of adductor SD. She experienced several viral upper respiratory infections where

the hoarseness associated with them did not go away. She was diagnosed by Dr. Elliott Morgan with the University of Alabama-Birmingham Otolaryngology department after a series of tests, including a CT scan, endoscopy, and videostroboscopy. She was offered Botox injections and had four treatments between September 2006 and April 2008. After the injections, she would lose her voice for about six weeks then would improve for up to six months. She met with a speech therapist who told her that voice therapy would not help and that she needed to accept her condition and continue Botox treatments. She found out about our approach through the website www.voicematters.net.

After reading my book, this patient contacted me with renewed hope that there was a way to recover from SD. She began working on the exercises in the book and enrolled in the January 2009 clinic. Her TJ profile was unremarkable. Her VHI was 71 (severe) and her fundamental frequency in connected speech was 189 Hz (low) with jitter 2.05 (very high) and shimmer 1.37 (high). She described speaking as a great effort, and that was obvious. She arrived at the clinic enthusiastic and ready for change. She had been praying and felt that God was leading her to the clinic to help her heal. She wanted her experience to be a testimony to His power in her life.

Highly compliant to all suggestions, her voice improved significantly at the clinic. She did well with easy onset, confidential voicing, pitch elevation, voicing with movement and breathing/chest expansion techniques. She was able to click into almost-normal voicing intermittently by the end of the week. Fundamental frequency of connected speech increased to 234 Hz, almost effortlessly. Upon her return home, she was able to practice daily and continued to report slipping in and out of her new groove. I met with her once when I was in her hometown and found her voice to be mostly smooth and flowing, with some voice breaks. Subjectively, her voice was moderately to significantly improved eight months after the clinic. The patient submitted the post-clinic paperwork. Her own assessment was that she had experienced significant improvement. Her VHI had decreased 24 points and was currently at 47 (moderate). She stated that her biggest problem was getting her new voice to work in public. She felt that in her home environment she was about 75 percent recovered, but when she was ordering food or interacting in other public situations, the voice would drop. I encouraged her to just keep re-grooving, and I have faith she will succeed completely.

I recently witnessed this patient's honest appraisal of her voice problems when I gave a talk to The Dystonia Society in her city. Prior to the talk she easily greeted me. Then, without warning, someone asked her to tell the group about her experience at the clinic and how it had helped. It was difficult for her to respond in a large group setting with no preparation. I could sense her panic. She had a few voice breaks but then stood up and used the body movement she had learned and increased breath and resonance to make an excellent adjustment. She is still moderately handicapped, but she is on the path to recovery. Many others fall in this category, possibly the majority of those we treat. More than 80 percent of those who return their feedback report moderate to significant improvements. The successes (normal to near-normal voice 90 percent or more of the time and no handicap) are on one end of the curve and failures (little to no improvement and possibly worsening condition) are at the other end, if the data are viewed as a bell curve. We have had some very complicated cases do very well. We have had fairly mild cases fail. SD recovery does not have a clear pattern of personality profile or even compliance. Length of time with the disorder does not necessarily denote chance of success. As has been noted repeatedly since this disorder was first described in the 1800s, it is a very puzzling and complex disorder; we have so much more to learn. With each success, there is hope.

Chapter 8
Intensive Post-Surgery Voice Rehabilitation

- **Case Study: Patient Q**

  Patient Q, a female pastor aged fifty, described gradual hoarseness beginning in fall 2001 during a stressful time. Her father passed away from amyotrophic lateral sclerosis (ALS), and she lost her voice. She described her voice at that time as strained, low, and cracking. She began speech therapy in 2002, which included laryngeal massage, but had no improvement in her voice. She was diagnosed with SD at the Mayo Clinic in Rochester, Minnesota. She tried Botox injections, which did help, with improvements lasting up to three months. She continued both Botox and speech therapy until January 2004, when she had Type II thyroplasty, with a stent placed between her vocal cords.

  The patient described that surgery as successful for three to four months, and she felt that the voice then "readjusted to sound like its former, strained self." Her physician, Dr. Nick Maragos, completed two additional surgeries in the spring of 2004 and 2005 to try to clear out tissue and muscles that seemed to interfere with vocal fold production. She experienced temporary improvement. She tried myofascial release, improved nutrition and hydration, and relaxation, and she began to use a soft voice with an amplifier. She was barely functioning at work. By 2006, she was working on just accepting the voice she had when she found out about the clinic on the internet. She enrolled January 2007.

Her TJ profile indicated that she was high in Depression, Anxiety, Inhibition, and Impulsivity. Acoustic analysis revealed a continuous speech fundamental frequency of 164 Hz (low), with jitter 4.9 (very high), and shimmer 2.3 (very high). Her VHI was 98 (severe). Subjectively, her voice was strained/pressed with considerable hoarseness. She was instructed in proper breathing techniques, relaxation techniques such as tongue and lip trills and humming. It was impossible for her to attain resonant voice, but given the stent in place and two additional surgeries, it was doubtful if completely normal voicing could be attained. This was discussed, as well as the possibility that she could learn a less effortful manner of voicing, moving the voice focus from her throat higher into the face, and lightening with a higher pitch and more inflection. With the vocal pitch elevated to 215 Hz, she felt little effort, and jitter decreased to .15 and shimmer to .5 (essentially normal). Six months later, she described moderate improvement, but her VHI, while significantly decreased, remained in the severe range. The patient continued to check in periodically and was continuing exercises until she was successful at incorporating strategies into daily conversational speech. More than two years after the clinic, I heard her voice on a Utube video, narrating a walk through the woods on snowshoes. Her voice sounded soft but smooth and effortless. I emailed her, and she completed follow-up once again. She sent the following testimonial, "The clinic in January 2007 was a turning point for me in feeling more control of my voice and my life. I think the surgeries were meant to re-groove my voice but it kept going back to what it knew. I learned ways at the clinic to re-groove my voice in a more holistic manner, bypassing the spasming voice and finding a new path to communication. It is more than the voice; it is a whole person thing. That includes an open, positive, attentive stance in relation to others. Through laughter, breathing, forgiveness, prayer, guided imagery, affirmations—I opened up to the possibility of healing on many levels." She reported significant improvement and stated that "a holistic, functional approach is the key to success." VHI had decreased to 43 (mild handicap).

- **Case Study: Patient R**

Patient R, a female, thirty-four presented with a lengthy and complicated history of voice problems starting at the age of ten. She remembered her voice quivering and breaking when speaking to her mother. She was diagnosed with stuttering, followed by years of speech therapy. At age eighteen, she married and resumed speech therapy. The treating speech therapist believed that she had SD, and she received an official diagnosis at Barnes Jewish Hospital in 1991. She received Botox injections every three to four months for several years. Initially, she would gain up to four months of improved voice that gradual declined. Then, the frequency of injections was increased to every two months. Eventually the benefit of the injections was limited to a few weeks. In 2003, her current ENT offered SLAD surgery, which she accepted. The results lasted for only one week before the spasms came back and her voice gradually worsened. In 2004, a stent was placed between the vocal folds. She was unable to speak for six months and when she did regain her voice, it was "spastic, hoarse, weak, and painful to produce."

At the time of the clinic, the patient estimated that she had had ninety-eight Botox injections in addition to the two surgeries. They no longer worked for her. The doctor had switched to Myobloc which is another variation of botulinum toxin, used when a person develops immunity to Botox. She found little relief. She was under the care of an ENT and a neurologist and was taking no medications. The patient was married with two children, ages eight and thirteen. She was currently active in church, exercise, and designing jewelry, in addition to her job as a physical therapy assistant. She reported a history of sexual, physical, and emotional abuse. She was extremely stressed over her chronic voice difficulties. Her TJ profile was very high in Nervousness (78th percentile), Depression (90th percentile), Inhibition, and Submissiveness.

She presented with a very high VHI score of 102. Acoustic analysis revealed a connected speech fundamental frequency of 156 Hz (low) with jitter 2.9 (high), and shimmer 1.0 (high). We targeted the emotional aspect of her difficulties extensively, as well as worked through strategies to increase her vocal range using sweeps with vowels. Release of effort, especially tightness in her abdominal musculature, and use of optimal breathing techniques were helpful. She was able to develop some increased resonance with a hum/speak method. By the end of the clinic, she had less hesitation and elevated her pitch to 175 Hz in connected speech. Following the clinic, with our encouragement, the patient sought out psychiatric care and started taking anti-anxiety and antidepressant medications. A phone consultation several months after the clinic confirmed her reports that her voice was improving. Seven months after the clinic, she reported moderately improved voice production, and a 44-point decrease in her VHI score, which took her from the Severe to Moderate range of handicap. It was very sad to me that this beautiful young woman had experienced so much pain and difficulty speaking her entire life. Recent emails indicate that she is maintaining her gains.

- **Case Study: Patient S**
Patient S, a female music teacher aged forty-eight, reported a history of vocal hoarseness dating back to 2000, when she was forty. She went to many doctors, who could not find the cause of her hoarseness. One doctor stated she had nodules and suggested surgery. A second opinion suggested she may have a unilateral vocal fold paralysis. In 2001, she went to Wake Forest University Medical Center for an evaluation with Dr. Gregory Postma. He conducted electromyography EMG studies as well as fiberoptic laryngoscopy and stroboscopy evaluations that confirmed a bilateral true vocal fold paresis. He suggested a unilateral medialization laryngoplasty. The patient was instructed that her voice should then be fine, or she might need surgery on the other side. He proceeded with a bilateral medialization with Gore-tex implants in June 2001.

Post-surgically, the patient was disappointed that her hoarseness continued. She was seen by several different speech therapists and improved somewhat. A follow-up evaluation with Dr. Potsma in August 2001 revealed "complete glottic closure with a good mucosal wave bilaterally. Left fold implant is prominent and medializes

the subglottis to some extent as well as a true vocal fold."
Voice therapy was recommended to address her occasional hyperfunctional episodes. She continued to work as a music teacher, using her voice extensively. She attended speech therapy intermittently but saw little improvement. The patient went to Nova Southeastern University in July 2004, and the report stated "moderate to severe hyperfunction characterized by medial compression of the ventricular folds and anterior-posterior compression during speech and phonation." This report made it clear that the patient was using her voice incorrectly, possibly as an attempt to speak with laryngeal structures altered by surgery.

The patient became depressed and anxious over the failure of her voice to improve. She was taking Effexor, which helped to control her emotional symptoms. She also took Prilosec for reflux. She was a self-described perfectionist who expected a lot from herself and her students. She had a very busy schedule with her classes (hundreds of students) as well as performance groups. She enrolled in the clinic in July 2007, hoping to learn new ways to use her voice without so much tension, and to improve her voice quality so she could teach more effectively in the coming school year. Patient S presented with a TJ high in Nervousness (71st percentile) and also high in Quiet and Inhibition. Her VHI was 86 (high). Acoustic analysis revealed fundamental frequency of connected speech of 169 Hz (low), with jitter 3.16 (very high), and shimmer 1.48 (high). Her breathing patterns were restricted and reversed. She was instructed to hum easily, reduce facial and jaw tension, use a kazoo, do lip and tongue trills, and perform all exercises prescribed to decrease the hyperfunction. Tension was evident throughout her body, but especially in her face, lips, tongue, throat, diaphragm, and abdominals. We discussed her anxiety over the upcoming school year and her difficulty in high voice use. She learned to release much of the tensions during the clinic, to connect the breath with the voice, and to increase her resonance. An elevation in pitch and use of increased airflow and intonation were helpful. By the end of the clinic, her perceived effort in voicing had decreased significantly.

We discussed the patient's disappointment with the surgery and how her efforts to produce an adequate voice were contributing to her problems. She had to learn to refocus her voice to produce more resonance. I recommended that she take a leave of absence from her job to establish more optimal and easy voice production. Since she lived several hours away, she came in for a session about once a month. She was compliant with her breathing and voice exercises and steadily improved. Seven months after the clinic, her feedback indicated a 40-point drop in her VHI, which placed her in the moderate category. She had established a pitch of 206 Hz, and jitter and shimmer both decreased. Strategies were discussed and put into place before she returned to work. I visited her at her school for a final session to do some role-playing in her actual teaching setting. At the school's initial open house, she received many comments from fellow teachers, parents, and students about how much better her voice sounded. She continues to be successful in her job during the second school year since the clinic. When the physical mechanism has been altered surgically, there is a limitation in what we can accomplish behaviorally. We try to be open and honest with these patients that we may not be able to help them achieve completely normal voicing when nerves have been altered or stents are in place. We have found that most are able to achieve significant improvements as we unravel compensatory behaviors associated with the physical sensations rendered by the structural changes and help them to maximize function.

Chapter 9
Failures?

In science and medicine, it is sometimes common for failures to be minimized or excluded. Those of us in the healing arts wish very much for all of our patients to experience success. I prefer full disclosure, and endeavor to present a complete overview of my patients' experiences. While it is the minority who found no significant benefit in the program, it was important to examine this. It was interesting to go over, first in my mind and then in my files, the people who I thought of as failing to demonstrate significant progress following the clinic. Maybe the clinic was not a good fit to their specific problems or their personality profiles. Perhaps it was not good timing. Perhaps the errant neurological activity was too great to overcome or re-groove. Perhaps there were psychological issues that were deeply repressed, and being unable to speak served some purpose that was not apparent. I had in mind those people who never sent feedback. Were they failures? The story of Patient O suggests that not all who benefit do so immediately, nor does failing to provide follow-up indicate that there has been no progress. "It takes as long as it takes" is my advice to all who try a holistic voice rehabilitation approach.

Since I can only report what I know to be true at the moment and rely on my patients to contact me with feedback, I don't know how accurate these "failures" will look in a year or two. I am not including those in the first year of rehabilitation because progress measured two to three years later seems to be more indicative of long-term success. Once people do experience success, it usually continues. Recovery may be slow at times or there may be setbacks, but there is a point when people recognize the control they have over their breathing, voice, and mind body, and there is no choice but to keep going forward. The key to true recovery is to avoid a panic response if it feels difficult to speak. I hope that these cases I am presenting as failures do not see themselves as failures but simply as still in recovery, and that they will find some way to be free to speak again, even if they do not attain vocal perfection.

- **Case Study: Patient T**

  Patient T, female, fifty-six, reported problems with her voice after an endoscopy in August 2004. It started as a weak voice and difficulty breathing. She was initially seen by an ENT, who prescribed Nexium and sent her to a speech therapist. She tried both the medication and the therapy for several months with no relief of symptoms. She visited a second ENT, who diagnosed her with adductor SD and arranged for her to go to Vanderbilt for Botox injections. She declined and continued to suffer from severe voice difficulties that affected her work with children and the elderly and put a strain on her social relationships and marriage. She was currently working as a house sitter, and her husband was retired.

  The patient described herself as an overly sensitive, nervous person. She was taking the antidepressant Effexor and blood pressure medication as well as over-the-counter acid reflux medication. She had problems with restless leg syndrome and sinus headaches. She had lost both her parents the previous year and her brother was in Iraq. Her VHI was 100 (severe) and her TJ profile indicated extreme

Anxious and Depressed symptoms. It was also high in Quiet, Inhibition, and Indifference, and relatively low in Self-Discipline. She attended the October 2006 clinic. Her pre-clinic homework questionnaire revealed struggles with self-discipline and low self-esteem as well as continued marital stress.

Acoustic analysis revealed fundamental frequency of 193 Hz (slightly low), jitter .28 (normal), and shimmer .54 (high). Subjectively, her voice was severely affected and it was challenging for her to speak. She did well with instructions to elevate her pitch to 200 to 225 Hz and to trigger deep breathing reflexes. She was able to hum easily and transfer that to words, phrases, and sentences. She left ecstatic and with the confidence that she had the tools to recover her voice totally. After several weeks, however, her communications with me stopped. She did not respond to requests for follow-up until almost a year after the clinic. She then reported that her voice had worsened (VHI had increased 14 points), and that she had been approximately 10 percent compliant to her contract. By completing the feedback, she realized that she was not practicing. She felt "embarrassed and ashamed" and recommitted herself to practicing what she needed to do. It has now been three years since the clinic, and I have not heard from the patient and do not know her current status.

- **Case Study: Patient U**

  Patient U, female, fifty-five was diagnosed with SD (unspecified type) by Dr. Jonathon Chinn in the spring of 2004. She had noticed that words were cutting out and, initially, voice therapy was recommended. Even after several months, voice therapy was unhelpful. The patient tried alternative therapies as well, including cranial-sacral treatments, hypnotherapy, and acupuncture. She joined a women's choir. She was taking no medications and had not tried Botox injections as a treatment. She described many stressors in her current life situation, including unemployment and family challenges. She attended the clinic in July 2007.

She presented with a VHI of 94 (severe). Her TJ profile was slightly above the norm for Nervous and Depressed, high in the Quiet and Inhibited categories, and high in Self-Discipline. Subjectively, her voice was extremely tight, cadence very slow, and effort high. She frequently experienced complete aphonia and was dysfluent. Fundamental frequency was 206 Hz (normal), jitter 1.4 (high), and shimmer .94 (high). However, when she spoke in unison and in imitation of short phrases, she could produce good voicing. Using a slightly higher pitch with attention to resonant voice was helpful. Singing practice helped her greatly, and she produced a lovely resonant singing voice at the clinic.

The patient did not stay in contact except for a brief phone consultation one month after the clinic and an email the next month. She was still experiencing a lot of difficulty but was encouraged as she found that she was managing her voice better overall. I did not hear from the patient until February 2009, nineteen months after the clinic. She said, "Sorry it has taken me so long. It has been hard to face my disappointment. I believe the work you are doing is good and do not want to discourage it. But for me, it did not work. I did my exercises religiously for 4 months and my voice continued to deteriorate. In January 2008, I tried Botox for the first time. It worked for two weeks during which I could speak softly and easily. Then my spasms returned and I began to speak on inhalation. I have now dropped the exhalation voice completely except when I practice. I tried Botox twice more, but it only gave me a sore throat. People tell me I sound better when I use inhalation voice, but I feel like I can't talk at all. It is like telling someone on crutches they are walking well. I also lost my ability to sing and had to leave the choir I love. I have not completely abandoned hope and try to keep listening for what the universe is offering." The follow-up VHI had increased 13 points.

- **Case Study: Patient V**

Patient V, female, sixty-three, described voice problems beginning in January 2006, gradually progressing over eighteen months to a swollen throat, voice breaks, and difficulty breathing. During this time, the patient worked in a medical office and had to talk on the phone or to patients for eight hours a day.

The patient saw three ENT doctors. Two diagnosed her with reflux and prescribed medications that did not help. A third diagnosed her with adductor SD. Speech therapy was recommended, but she did not go, except to see Morton Cooper for a four-hour consultation. She had been working with his strategies as well as those listed in my first book. She had also tried acupuncture, herbal treatments, structural energetic therapy, chiropractic, and acupressure. Her only medication was Armour Thyroid, and she had not tried Botox treatments.

She attended the clinic in July 2007. VHI was 73 (severe) and her TJ profile was remarkable for high scores in Submissiveness and Impulsivity. In her session with the psychologist, she reported that she often felt like she "did not have a voice" and had problems setting boundaries with others. Incidentally, she reported that her mother had an SD-like voice but, at the age of eighty-four, had never been diagnosed or treated. The patient was married with three adult daughters and nine grandchildren, active in her church, gardening, art tours, jazzercise, and walking. In addition to her full-time job, she was also helping her husband with a book project.

Acoustic analysis revealed a fundamental frequency of 165 Hz (low), jitter 1.3 (high), and shimmer .98 (high). A natural hum and instant voice press indicated a resonant tone between 220 and 250Hz, and she had an excellent range of two and a half octaves. Focus was mostly in her throat although she had been trying to practice humming with facial focus. She was using confidential voice with fair success. The breathing coach worked with her extensively to open up the channel for her breath, which had become restricted. The first eight months after the clinic, she stayed in contact frequently. She had gone on disability and was unemployed most of that time, so she had ample time to participant in voice rehabilitation. She felt that she maintained her compliance contract at about 80 percent, and she continued her search for various methods that might help her voice. She enrolled in yoga, Feldenkreis lessons, and Low Energy Neurofeedback treatments. None helped her voice.

After six to eight months, the patient indicated that her voice was no better and possibly even worse than before the clinic. VHI had increased to 86. Despite the lack of improvement, she stated that the clinic was well conceived and quite helpful. She continued working on her voice and was able to access it on occasion. More than two years after the clinic, she stated, "I am in the failure category, but I have hope of a miracle one day. I have been unemployed for years due to my voice, but recently found a job with the help of a county service for people with disabilities. I enjoy it and do not have to talk constantly. Unfortunately, I do not have any good voice days and sometimes I can't even get one word out. Despite it all, I have remained cheerful, happy, and enjoy my life and the people in it. I feel healthy with lots of energy. I just sound different. I found the clinic very worthwhile and would recommend it." I suggested that she might wish to explore Botox as a possible treatment at this point.

- **Case Study: Patient W**

Patient W, a male elementary school teacher aged forty-three, began having trouble with his voice in March 2007, during his divorce from his wife of eighteen years. His voice "cut in and out when speaking loudly," and it steadily worsened over a ten-month period. In December, an ENT diagnosed him with MTD or SD and recommended speech therapy. He had three sessions of therapy, during which the therapists determined they did not know how to treat his condition. He met with Dr. Robert Bastion in February 2008, who confirmed a diagnosis of abductor SD. He was given a .7 u shot of Botox, an injection of 1.7 u ten days later, and a third injection of 3u two months following the second one. The patient stated that none of the injections improved his voice, only resulting in noisy inhalation.

The patient was taking no medications and had not tried any alternative treatments at the time of the clinic. He presented with a VHI of 104 (severe), and while he rated the importance of voice recovery very high, he was concerned about emotional issues and his strong personality working against him in his efforts. He said he had difficulty with change and always had a hard time breaking out of a routine. His wife had suggested the divorce and was involved with someone else. He would have custody of his son, while she would have custody of their two daughters. He felt his sisters were supporting his ex-wife. He had a lot of stress around the time he lost his voice, and he could pinpoint the month that it happened; his sisters went on vacation with his ex-wife and her boyfriend. He was also having trouble teaching at the time regarding disciplining his students or speaking up. At the initial evaluation, the patient stated that he would like to recover his voice to be an effective teacher and parent, and to communicate to be able to find a new life-partner.

The patient's TJ was unremarkable with the exception of a high score in Inhibition. Despite his current situation, he did not appear highly anxious or depressed and was Self-Disciplined (98th percentile). Acoustic analysis revealed fundamental frequency of 136 Hz (slightly high), jitter 2.4 (high), and shimmer 1.3 (high). He was able to produce almost two octaves on a vowel. He did not report excessive effort on speaking, but had considerable nasal air flow during speaking and was often aphonic. He appeared to push through speaking from an abdominal focus.

The patient was trained on Voiceprint so he could view his pitch and resonance. The voice press revealed that a lower pitch was optimal (100 to 115 Hz) to produce resonant voice. Production of "er" was good, and the patient demonstrated his ability to engage the vocal folds for good vocalization. The patient often stated that he had given up on his voice, and he seemed disconnected from the new good voice that he was capable of. Throughout the week, he was able to click into the new voice intermittently. At times, he became easily conversational but then would struggle once more. His post-analysis at the end of the week was virtually unchanged.

At the six-month follow-up, the patient described no change in his voice except that it was slightly better on occasion. He stated that he was about 20 percent compliant with the program and had not viewed his DVD of the clinic. He felt that an even more intensive program with more one-to-one contact in voice and psychological counseling would have been beneficial. He described putting more effort into the program and that his voice had returned for about a month, but it slipped away. He got a glimpse of what it felt like to be free to speak, but it was short-lived. He indicated that he was using the exercises but still had "no voice." We suggested that he revisit psychological consultation or voice therapy or both. As of our last communication, he had not followed up with a psychologist or voice therapist, and he was no longer teaching but was working in a technology job that decreased the need for voice use.

Chapter 10
Private Consultations

It is not always possible for patients to take the time and money to attend an intensive clinic, so I also offer private voice therapy for SD clients. If they are from another state or country, I recommend a minimum of three hours' consultation, and I make a DVD so that I can assess them and teach them as much as I can while providing them a tool for follow-up. As I reported with the patients who participate in the intensive clinics, some continue to follow up with me over a number of years, periodically checking in with a visit or a phone consultation, while others do not contact me after the first consultation. I can only report on those who provide follow-up information. I find that most people who fall in this category try a variety of approaches that contribute to their successes. I might play only a small part in that, but I do offer hope and direction, even when my time with them is limited.

- **Case Study: Patient X**
  Patient X, female, thirty-six, reported difficulties beginning at the birth of her son, six years prior to the consultation. She was finally diagnosed with SD in Wokingham, UK, after taking beta blocker medication for stress, undergoing speech therapy, and visiting various physicians for four years. She was diagnosed with mixed SD at Oxford Radcliffe Hospital. Botulinum toxin injections were rec-

ommended, but she declined. I saw her for a three-hour consultation in June 2008.

The patient was currently not taking medication and was having upper body massage therapy every six weeks. She reported that her voice caused her stress in her family relationships and in her full-time job as a general manager/director. She reported great inconsistency in her voice on a daily basis, including good voice production that suddenly "sounds terrible," and she said she was unable to talk on the telephone. Her VHI score was 83 (severe). Subjectively, she presented with symptoms of primarily abductor SD.

Acoustic analysis revealed a fundamental frequency of 186 Hz (low), with jitter and shimmer both at 1.1 (high). She felt a definite effort in speaking most of the time. Her breathing pattern was reversed. Her natural hum was at 232 Hz so she was instructed to pitch her voice higher. Yoga was recommended as she was very tight, especially in the area of the chest and diaphragm and I felt that it might help her improve her breathing patterns. We discussed phone strategies and practiced them. The patient was over-thinking the problems, which caused more tension and anxiety around speaking. She was instructed to shift from over-thinking her problem to sensing and feeling her breathing and voice flow. We also discussed and practiced resonant voice therapy strategies. She was instructed to "groove in" the difficult consonants such as "h" and "s," beginning with single words and progressing as she felt confident.

Other than a brief email, the patient did not contact me until recently. In October 2009, sixteen months after the consultation, she reported, "My voice has improved dramatically. I cut out caffeine completely. I exercise more regularly and possibly by gaining confidence in my appearance and spreading endorphins around, my voice has been transformed. The breathing control together with thinking positively has helped. I have my odd days, but by calming myself and doing something positive, my voice improves. Many people have commented lately on how my voice has improved and some ask if I actually even have a voice problem. I really do think that in my case, how I am feeling and thinking can cause my voice to deteriorate. When I am feeling most relaxed and socializing, my voice is good." Her VHI had decreased 48 points, putting her in the mild handicap range with a total score of 35.

- **Case Study: Patient Y**

  Patient Y, female, fifty-one, reported voice difficulties dating back to August 2000 when her voice began to slowly deteriorate. She reported significant trauma associated with the onset of full-blown SD in 2001. She supplied medical documentation of her problems in 2001, where she reported voice difficulties and was referred to an ENT. She later developed chest pains and reflux and her voice became more strained. She had a previous diagnosis of irritable bowel syndrome. Her doctor initially thought that her voice problems were related to reflux and recommended Prilosec. Medical records also documented voice complaints in 2002. That December, she saw a neurologist who suspected SD. Dr. Timothy Anderson at the Lahey Clinic confirmed the diagnosis of SD in February 2003.

  The patient tried speech therapy as well as Botox three times. She felt that the results were not sufficient to continue the injections, so she researched and found Dr. Cooper's website. Since Dr. Anderson was well aware that Botox was not working for her, he wrote a letter of recommendation that she try Dr. Cooper's DVR. Surgery was the only other option he could offer her at the time. This was in February 2005. The patient immediately scheduled an appointment and spent four weeks with Dr. Cooper. She experienced improvement and developed a stronger voice while there but quickly deteriorated when she returned home. She stated that she practiced three times daily for eighteen months but continued to struggle with basic conversations. The patient contacted me by email in 2006. She expressed feeling very guilty about spending a great deal of her time and money with Dr. Cooper and not being able to maintain her gains or continue to progress. She was considering our clinic but was unable to afford it. She had adult children living at home, problems with in-laws, a full-time job, and chronic stress. She was on medications for hypothyroidism and estrogen replacement. Well aware that breathing was an issue for her, she ordered the recommended DVD from Mike and started his optimal breathing development program on her own. We emailed back and forth, and I made suggestions, but I needed more input to assess and guide her. She was able to schedule a three-hour consultation with me in February 2007.

The patient's VHI was 106 (very high). Acoustic analysis was mostly average, with fundamental frequency of continuous speech at 215 Hz, jitter at .5, and shimmer at 1.8. She spoke in a very slow rate with a staccato or hard glottal attack on most words. It took her twice the average time to read the first two sentences of the phonetically balanced Rainbow Passage that I use in my analysis of connected speech. She had great difficulty humming, with tension and focus in the throat. She pushed from her abdominals, causing vocal arrest (similar to what occurs in the Valsalva maneuver when one holds the breath). The holding back of the breath causes the vocal folds to push together, stopping their vibration. She also tended to bob her head as she spoke. We worked on movement with sound to develop more of a flow, singing practice with the Roger Love CD, lip and tongue trills, and a lot of sensing/feeling the voice because she was over-thinking it. Work with "m" words and phrases to help pull the focus forward out of the throat were prescribed.

A follow-up phone consultation in April 2007 indicated some improvement but continued chronic stress and anxiety. Mental health counseling and possible medication were discussed. In May 2007, the patient began massage therapy, an exercise program, and a mild antidepressant/anti-anxiety medication. We lost touch for a while, but I received an email from her in June 2009. She stated that she was slowly improving on her voice production. She was still feeling overly stressed, working long hours. She had discontinued her antidepressant medication after a year. Follow-up in October 2009, two and a half years after the initial consultation and three years after our initial email conversations, she stated that she was continuing to improve slowly and knew that she needed more time for herself. The breathing exercises were helpful as she was moving out of the staccato manner of speech into more of a flow. She provided an updated VHI, which indicated a 41-point decrease since the initial consultation. Her score was 65, which is low severe.

The patient stated that she attributed her improvement to what she learned from her month with Dr. Cooper, my book and our consultation, voice lessons with Alma Veja, work with a talented massage therapist, meeting and talking with others who had overcome SD, and breathing techniques. I wish her well on this long, difficult journey, and I am glad to have made some contribution.

- **Case Study: Patient Z**

  Patient Z, male, fifty-three, reported voice difficulties beginning in spring 2004 following a throat infection. Initially, he was told he had edema in the vocal folds and was treated medically for that. Over the next two years, his voice slowly deteriorated. The ENT could find nothing wrong, so he was referred for psychiatric treatment and given anti-anxiety medication. After eight months with the voice not improving, the patient had a series of tests, and a neurologist diagnosed him with SD in October 2005. He had his first botulinum toxin injection in January 2006. The patient declared it a complete success in that his voice improved immediately and lasted for eight months. The second injection gave him no relief of symptoms. He contacted me in May 2008 and we arranged a consultation during my next trip to London. We arranged for a five-hour consultation in June 2008.

  He presented with a VHI of 74 (severe). He had purchased Mike's breathing DVD and had begun practicing with it. Acoustic analysis revealed a connected speech fundamental frequency of 129 Hz (normal), with slightly elevated jitter and shimmer. Voice production and speech was quite effortful. Focus was mainly in the throat. A slightly lower pitch was optimal (118 to 128 Hz), but the focus needed to move upward into the face. He did well with lip and tongue trills and use of a confidential voice with no push. His abdominals were extremely tight, restricting a free flow of the breath. There was a lot of tension in the muscles of the neck, which tended to pull the larynx high in the neck. We worked on low larynx exercises and resonant voice techniques. He did well working with "h" words and phrases to release more air through the glottis.

The patient played soccer and worked a lot, with no planned relaxation in his schedule. He was divorced with three adult children, working full-time as a real estate agent in Spain. Due to the economic downturn, work had become very stressful. We discussed the importance of relaxation and developing the parasympathetic nervous system. He agreed to explore yoga or Tai Chi, massage, Alexander technique, and other forms of grounding and centering himself to reduce stress and anxiety.

The patient kept in touch with me regularly, and we met again in February 2009. His pitch had actually increased based on the acoustic analysis, but effort had decreased slightly. At that time, VHI had decreased 21 points and was in the moderate range at 53. He had been trying a variety of approaches to manage his stress and improve his voice, including homeopathic treatments, Shiatsu, Tai Chi, reflexive meditation, and reflexology. He continued to express fear around speaking situations but was recognizing the fear and learning to control his stress level and relax. He found that, "If I speak more loudly in a bold way, the voice is better."

Six months later, the patient reported, "Since I met you, my voice has improved significantly. It is so important to have expert advice, but to have it from an expert who has experienced the problem firsthand is something more. I still have days that I let the stress get to me, but most of the time I feel I have made great progress. I realize I am letting others stress me out. I get on Voiceprint and do some Roger Love sounds, think and say positive things to myself, and then my voice becomes good again. I still need to master relaxing my stomach muscles in order to be 'in control' of my voice, as you obviously are. I'm sure I will get there eventually." He continues to keep in touch and to progress.

Chapter 11

Can Holistic Voice Rehabilitation Become an Accepted Option?

I have mentioned some of the skepticism and criticism of our program to date. As with the introduction of most novel ideas, there follows either unhealthy refusal to consider it or healthy examination of the process. The need for better treatment outcomes for SD is clearly voiced over and again. But change is often unwelcome. Botox is the gold standard and, for many professionals, that is enough to keep prescribing it and remain adamant that it is the best treatment we have. It is easier to stay "in the box," and many scientists would argue that we must stay in that box until another method is scientifically proven. Some of the problems with scientific rigor have already been discussed.

Holistic voice rehabilitation takes a voice problem and treats it as a whole mind body problem. Dr. John Sarno described holistic as a treatment *considering both the emotional and structural aspects* of a disorder. He made the point that it does *not reject the scientific method.* Although he is a medical physician and professor, with vastly broader training and experience than I, his writings and journal proposals were almost universally denied publication within the field because his concepts of holistic treatment fly in the face of contemporary medical dogma. Hence, he published books from 1984 to 2006.

I was introduced to Dr. Sarno's work on psychosomatic disorders after the publication of my first book. I was asked to conduct a seminar on my approach to SD to a group of Canadian Speech Pathologists. During the question and answer session, I was asked if I had patterned my approach after Dr. Sarno. I regrettably had never read any of his books. However, I began that week. Born in 1923, Dr. Sarno has been affiliated with the New York University School of Medicine since the 1960s. He primarily worked in rehabilitation medicine and discovered that many pain syndromes could be managed by working through underlying emotional issues. Some mistake this to mean problems are purely psychological, yet Dr. Sarno explains that the physical manifestation is very real. He includes in this group of disorders not only pain syndromes, but gastric reflux, peptic ulcer, larnygospasm, irritable bowel, tension and migraine headaches, sexual dysfunction, carpal tunnel syndrome, and fibromyalgia. Modern medicine has pharmaceutical or surgical treatments for all of these, but modern medicine does not seem to recognize or discuss the emotional possibilities as an important part of the whole.

A pioneer in the field, Dr. Sarno has many followers. His latest book, *The Divided Mind: The Epidemic of Mindbody Disorders* (2006), is an excellent exploration, with chapters by other leading physicians. In the introduction, even after four decades of successfully treating patients, Dr. Sarno states, "I undoubtedly will be challenged by the guardians of perceived wisdom for the so-called lack of scientific evidence for my diagnostic theories. This is almost ludicrous since there is no scientific evidence for some of the most cherished conventional concepts of symptom causation." Fifteen years earlier, his book *Healing Back Pain* (1991) was a New York Times Best-seller. Those suffering with back pain were more interested in relief than scientific evidence and acceptance.

I am not in the league of Dr. John Sarno, but that a man of his distinction was denied publication in medical journals and scorned by many of his fellow physicians helps me to be brave in the face of those who stand against my attempts to present a new solution to a serious voice condition. Also, when my voice begins to weaken, I know how to use my emotions and the power of my mind to move back into the right groove. I can teach others to do the same. More importantly, it helps me be realistic about the possibility that the professional majority may never accept this approach and see clearly that it is not necessary to be recognized and "scientifically proven" to help others.

Most of the elite voice specialists, those who have earned doctoral degrees and published research papers, advise me that I must engage in proper scientific research. This advice is universal, and not only from critics. I started a file of data from the beginning, with the intention of submitting a formal paper to one of the respected journals. I found it to be an arduous task, and upon further investigation as to the requirements, I did not feel that I could adequately compose a scientific paper. Most journal editors are looking for higher educational qualifications from their authors, specifically a PhD. I was having difficulty describing voice rehabilitation in scientific terms. The more anxiety I felt over trying to "prove" myself and this approach to the scientific world, the worse I felt internally. I let self-doubt and frustrations build until, not surprisingly, my voice began to suffer. My voice is such a wonderful indicator for my internal state. I abandoned that project for the purpose of completing this book and becoming free to speak once more!

I now know that providing proof may not be possible, at least within the scientific model. The theoretical focus, eclectic principles, and holistic nature of the program simply do not

- 109 -

allow purely scientific study. I understand the hesitancy of the professional community to collaborate, but I want to make it clear that my intention is to share what I know about helping broken voices, and that this book is part of that intention. Even discussions about needing a control group upset me greatly. How could I offer some sham treatment when I have knowledge that can truly help someone move beyond SD and gain more power and control? I cannot stop offering to help others overcome SD. If holistic voice rehabilitation remains "outside the box," then I must be content with that. It need not replace Botox, as there will always be those who choose or need that treatment. But with the preliminary data that more than 80 percent of people who used my method have significantly improved voices, more personal control, and less handicap, the proof is there.

If you are suffering from SD or treating those who have it, do not be afraid of becoming, in the words of world-renowned, award-winning writer Paulo Coelho, a "Warrior of the Light." His book by that title consists of short notes on accepting failure, embracing life, and rising to your destiny. Every person who overcomes SD and becomes free to speak is a beacon of light for the next. Every success of voice rehabilitation and recovery of functional voicing extends power for the next generation of SD sufferers.

New ideas need space. Body and soul need new challenges. The future has become the present, and every dream—except those dreams that involve preconceived ideas—will have a chance to be heard. In order to have faith in his own path, (the Warrior) does not need to prove that someone else's path is wrong.—Paulo Coelho

Chapter 12
Basic Principles of Holistic Intensive Voice Rehabilitation

Accept the Responsibility for Change

The primary idea behind voice rehabilitation as I view it is to help a person develop self-responsibility for changing voice production and moving beyond the SD voice. Although people may accept treatment through other modalities, medical or alternative or both, they need to realize that ultimate change comes from within. No one chooses to get SD. Whether it comes on slowly or suddenly, it is a terrible affliction and changes a person's life. It is easy to feel victimized and helpless because easy voice production is in the past, making a person feel out of control.

The out-of-control feeling may be because voice production is largely an automatic process, much like walking or breathing. Voice production, especially for the purpose of communication via language, is regulated in the brain in complex ways we don't yet understand. The autonomic nervous system plays a role, but the interplay of sensory (feeling) and motor (action) input to and from the brain via the vagus nerve, along with our auditory feedback, emotion, and cognition all play a part. It is not surprising that something along this long and winding path can go wrong and produce an undesirable result. Then, because of the automatic nature of voice production, the voice probably gets off groove somewhere along the way, causing changes in brain activity to have a negative impact.

We have to, for a time, become aware of how we are using our voices. The degree to which a person can take control and make changes is variable. The process begins with examining what may have led to the initial voice changes and knowing how intricately the emotions and the voice are connected. Because the causes of SD are numerous and complex, this is not an easy task. One must examine commitment to the process as well as any significant factors that might be interfering with the process. A person is encouraged to accept the voice as it is but know that it can be changed. If someone cannot embrace the idea of actually being in control of his or her voice, voice rehabilitation will be in vain. The first step is to accept a certain degree of control in order to move from automatic to regulated voice production. Once habituated, a new automatic process can be established. The new automatic process is demonstrated when people who stutter become fluent and in people who change accents or articulatory behaviors.

Another example of changing an automatic process comes to mind. I have worked with many teenagers and adults who exhibited tongue thrust while swallowing. Most came to see me because their orthodontic procedures were in vain; they continued to have an overbite/overjet despite lengthy treatment because of their swallow pattern. They were pushing their tongues against their front teeth when they swallowed, hundreds of times a day. Swallowing is fairly automatic. We don't think, "Oh, I must swallow by placing my tongue at the alveolar ridge behind my teeth, pressing there, elevating my larynx, closing it off so I don't choke," and so forth. We simply swallow. But in about thirteen weeks, most people with average cognitive abilities can learn to re-pattern the swallow. Exploratory motor learning is key in the process, and with daily practice and bringing awareness to swallowing, a new automatic is created. I believe this same motor learning can aid in voice recovery.

Next, a channel for the natural voice must be established and re-grooved. A person must learn to pay attention to all the sub-systems of voice production and fine-tune them. By slipping into a different groove repetitively, and with practice and strategies, changes can and do happen! The emphasis is on letting go of the gripping mind and anxiety around the voice and beginning to sense and feel the natural voice emerging. Almost every person with SD has a "good voice," which may be humming, singing, talking to pets or young children, talking to themselves in the shower, using a foreign accent, or speaking upon awakening from sleep. They must access *the good voice* and groove that in. Numerous methods facilitate re-grooving.

Basic Target Areas of Exploration

As with any good voice therapy program, our program aims to coordinate the breathing, pitch, focus, and resonance in a fluid, non-restricted manner. We work on voice image and psychological blocks, exploring contributing factors in a person's life and self-image issues. It involves taking control over the problem by transforming an automatic reflexive type of voice into one that is volitional to find a new groove. The following are crucial aspects of holistic voice rehabilitation. Specific exercises are covered in Chapter 15.

A. Psychological Aspects: Mental Preparation

Mental preparation is the basis for all cognitive-behavioral changes. People must accept their personal power and gain a sense of control over their situations. With SD, most people have been told there is nothing to do but get a shot and learn to live with the treatments. Setting the stage for success by committing to a process that will likely take time to accomplish is an important beginning.

It is necessary for every client to explore the emotions around communicating and the history of the voice issues. They need to explore self-image, self-worth, self-acceptance, and their ideas around being "free to speak." Psychological factors exist in a large number of those diagnosed with SD, which could be the primary etiology or a result of living with a broken voice. Recently, as the keynote speaker at the 2010 Voice Symposium, Robert Sataloff, MD, stated, "Our SD patients do not have SD because they are crazy; they are crazy because of the SD." This is a poignant statement that we need to keep in perspective.

However, if people's subconscious minds tell them they have no right to a voice, no power to express their inner feelings, their bodies may stay locked in that state. In the cases of severe depression, anxiety, or mood disorders, medications can be helpful for a short time, perhaps a year or more, to help stabilize the emotions and reestablish a sense of calm acceptance. Others use acupuncture, herbal treatments, or other alternative methods to help in this area. Psychological counseling can also be a huge benefit.

Because we conduct psychosocial testing prior to the clinic, I have found that approximately 80 percent of those we see score high in Anxiety and Depression. Inhibition is also frequently high. Again, whether these were contributing factors to the voice problem or the result of it is the big question. Either way, we spend quite a bit of time exploring the psychological history and progression of the voice problem. Often, people recognize that they have a history of "not being heard," being "unable to speak out and express themselves safely," or other factors. They realize how these ideas have been reinforced by SD. Avoidance behaviors play into the mix as well. No program that addresses simply the mechanical aspects of voice production is likely to help those with SD.

Loss of voice or serious voice dysfunction that may be diagnosed as SD is occasionally the result of a psychological "conversion" disorder. The prognosis for this type of voice dysfunction is excellent, and rapid complete voice return can quickly occur once the emotions behind it are processed. In other cases, there are such deep emotional scars that appear to be so painful that the conscious mind is unable to process them. The mind chooses a physical symptom to distract it from what is too painful to recognize and accept. I've heard stories of incest, abuse, and tragedies voiced for the first time in my office. Issues such as these, so deeply woven into a person's being, precede voice dysfunction by many years and can keep one seriously "armored" and unable to move forward with any significant life change. In other cases, a person may subconsciously have some secondary benefit from the voice dysfunction, and the recovery of the voice may not serve them as well as being unable to speak. These people are not crazy, and it is not a simple task to unravel the emotions from the actual physical symptoms of the voice disorder.

B. *Whole Body Work*

In our treatment program, we borrow from the creative arts and from the bodywork of various disciplines. We apply whole body work since we recognize that the voice is more than just a mix of laryngeal muscles operating from a set of cortical controls in the brain. Use of body alignment and movement is crucial to releasing the true, free voice. Much of what we use comes from the Alexander technique. F.M. Alexander, born in 1869, was a Shakespearian actor with bouts of voice loss, and no doctor in his day could help him to resolve it. He set out to find for himself what the problem was and began a practice of self-observation. He discovered his own "misuse" of his body and voice, eventually correcting it. He set out to *inhibit habitual patterns that interfered with voice production.* This involved a high level of consciousness of the total self. He developed a technique that balanced strength, coordination, and ease of movement using dynamic pose and changing habits of thought and movement. The Alexander technique is brilliant. He taught in London and occasionally in the U.S. until 1955. His technique lives on in the hands of his students and followers.

Although I have only a brief introduction to Feldenkrais bodywork, many people also find these techniques helpful in developing better body awareness and efficiency of breathing and movement. I've had reports from people suffering with SD who have improved their voice use through Feldenkrais lessons. *Freeing the Natural Voice* (Linklater 2006) is another resource of exercises aimed at unlocking "intellectual blocks, aural blocks, and psychological blocks" to free the voice by freeing the whole person.

We find that body explorations can quickly cut through and change perception and production in the voice. We often employ body movement and may be found "breast stroking" around the room as we speak or "picking apples," altering held postures that free us up and help us recognize our habitual holding patterns. Some patterns keep us stuck, and we develop a new intention of unlocking and moving to a new way of being. Some aspects of yoga are innately helpful, not only in improving the psyche and brain chemistry, but also in opening up the entire physical body, making more room for breath and voice. There are postures that help us attain this; in yoga, these are shoulder, chest, thoracic spine, and hip opening poses. Yoga practice often uses the chakra system, or energy centers in the body, which can be helpful in opening up the breath and the voice. Although most speech therapists use sitting in a chair as standard practice for conducting therapy, this may not be the best position for exploring the voice.

General relaxation is very important. In my first book, I described Jacobson's Progressive Relaxation technique. It has a history of success since 1930 and consists of progressively tensing and releasing specific muscles of the body to lead to total relaxation. However, a multitude of excellent guided imagery and relaxation techniques are now available on CD or DVD. I find that the relaxation achieved while being guided by a soothing voice set to music is incredibly valuable. One suggestion is *Psychosomatic Wellness; Healing your Bodymind* (2004) by Candace Pert, PhD, which includes scientifically based meditation set to music. Numerous choices are available based on different personal or spiritual paths. My yoga practice offers a beginning and ending shavasana, which is a mindful meditation, letting go of all tensions, both mental and physical. The main objective is to allow oneself to do nothing but surrender the body mind. We so seldom allow ourselves this opportunity. Sleep is not an alternative for a period of purposeful awareness in deep relaxation that has amazing healing potential.

C.   *Breathing for Speech*

Much of what I originally learned about breathing came from the research of Michael White. He is rather a breathing guru, since he spent much of the past thirty years exploring the topic and developing Optimal Breathing. His website, born of his passion and research, is a plethora of information on assessing and teaching correct breathing techniques. Although Michael no longer provides the breathing development services for the clinics, his contributions are invaluable (Optimal Breathing® and Breathing.com. Copyright © Michael White 2006, 2008). It has been very interesting to find that most voice therapy books and what people have learned from well-meaning voice specialists is contrary to what is needed for connecting the breath to the voice. Breathing is given more attention in the world of singers, but breathing for singing and for speech is not the same. Almost every person with SD has poor breath control. Their ways of using the breath interfere with good voice production.

Which comes first, poor voice production or poor breath control? This is a good question, and it may be either situation in different people. I do know that when one has SD, breathing becomes dysfunctional and restricted. It is common to have complaints such as, "I feel like I don't have enough breath to speak with," or "I feel as if I am holding my breath while I speak." There is most definitely a disconnection with the flow of breathing and the production of voice. There may be too little or too much airflow or a combination of the two. The person with SD or voice dysfunction must connect with the core of the breathing. The dysfunction needs to be uncovered and the breathing must first become deeper and unimpeded. Then the voice must be added so that it rides out on the breath. As with the voice, breathing patterns are automatic in the mindbody, and dysfunctional patterns must be re-trained. One of the most common errors that voice therapists make is to tell people they need to pull the abdominal muscles inward for voice production. This is contraindicated for those with SD, who instinctively use excessive abdominal "push" to get the voice out. This, instead, blocks the voice and can result in a voice break or arrest in AD/SD patients or a breathy break or rush of air in AB/SD patients. A slight push outward while vocalizing can be quite freeing. A connection with the core of one's being is needed. An inhalation should move downward toward the belly, allowing the belly to become soft and move outward. Once the inhalation is complete and the belly has moved outward as a result of the diaphragm moving downward as the lungs inflate, voice can begin as a passive force, not an active force. Voice is produced by a small amount of air during exhalation and should never be forced. A slight push out of the belly allows this passive action to occur, and voice production often becomes easier as the tendency to use abdominal strength to try to control the vocal folds diminishes.

For a basic exploration of the breath, put one hand on your chest and one on your abdomen. Breathe naturally.

Feel what is happening. Which hand rises on the inhale? If it is the abdomen, you are at least on target. If you feel no movement in the abdomen or a depression on the inhale, you need to seriously re-pattern your breathing pattern. Your rate of breathing is also important. If you are breathing at a fast rate, every two to four seconds, for example, there is a problem. You should slowly inhale for at least six to eight seconds and then slowly exhale for slightly longer, followed by a pause before the next inhalation. According to research, slowing one's habitual breath rate is a significant indicator for overall health.

I also learned in Hatha yoga practice how inward rotation of my shoulders and collapsed thoracic spine impeded my breath flow. As I have opened up in these areas, breathing and voicing are much easier. With SD, my diaphragm was locked up and did not allow a full movement of breath that triggered the movement of my body. Study of the Alexander technique allowed me to explore how poor habits of movement were impeding my breath and my voice. The clinic's current breathing coach, Dennis Price, is skilled at neuromuscular therapy and can quickly break through limiting muscle tension anywhere in the body.

Breathing is not as simple as we might think. It is not only the in-and-out of air through our lungs. It can be helpful to visualize the depth and breadth of air as if it flowed through the whole body. Of course, it doesn't, but in order to fill the lungs fully, the diaphragm must be free to move down on the inhalation, which is then felt as a larger space in the stomach, sides, and back. The breath can become much deeper than we might imagine. The diaphragm must be free to move downward on the inhalation. If not, we may experience a panic reaction, the Valsalva maneuver, which locks the diaphragm and does not allow proper breathing. The abnormal voice production observed in SD and any related disorder is commonly associated with the abnormal breath support or constriction of breath that occurs with the Valsalva maneuver. Simply gasp in quickly as if a man with a gun just burst through your door, and you will experience this phenomenon. It is impossible to speak when you are in this state. A release of the diaphragm lock is necessary for the breath and voice to flow. This Valsalva hypothesis has been implicated and discussed in the case of stuttering (Parry 2006), and I believe it plays a role in many cases of SD as well.

D. *Voice Development: Focus, Resonance, and Pitch*

One of the first things to assess and target is the proper focus of the voice. Most people with SD focus the voice deep in the throat and produce voice with great effort. The voice lacks any resonance. This is because the resonating cavities of the throat, palate, and oral and nasal cavities are not being utilized. The voice gets "stuck" in the throat. If you can hum easily and freely and the sound produced is "felt" as vibrations along the upper palate and into the nose and cheeks, it is an indication that your vocal folds can vibrate normally. You need to use that hum to place the voice. I like to call that the *anchor*. Initially, lots of humming is encouraged. If a hum is not possible, this is usually due to some restriction in the vocal tract, extreme tension of the solar plexus, diaphragm, or abdomen, or in the muscles of the tongue, palate, pharynx, or neck. The vocal folds may be pushing too tightly or pulling apart but, keep in mind, there is nothing wrong with the vocal folds themselves. It is their activity that is amiss, misdirected by signals from the brain. A key feature of SD is that the actual vocal folds appear normal. It is their movement that is abnormal or inconsistent.

People with SD often have a muscular tension overlay, postural problems such as mal-alignment of the spine with the head too far forward or back, a hunched posture with inward rotation of the shoulders and collapse of the upper torso, or a panic response when attempting vocalization, which shuts down the flow of air to some degree with a tightening of the solar plexus.

If you are humming yet feel the vibrations in the throat, you are not making use of your resonators. Sometimes a sincere *mmm-hmm*, as if agreeing with someone, helps to place the hum more resonantly. At times it is necessary to get the breathing patterns corrected before a resonant hum can be produced. Certainly posture and unraveling physical tension in the body and anxiety around using the voice are equally important. If a person has anticipatory anxiety, which is fear upon speaking, it will affect the end result of vocalization. One must let go of the gripping mind and the gripping muscles that interfere with vocal fold movement.

Humming is often the first step in the recovery process, and it is of utmost importance. Humming can help a person move into chanting using syllables with "m" or "n" words and, eventually, into hum-speaking, where an entire sentence is "hummed" while spoken silently. Then the same sentence is spoken aloud as the person attempts to keep the resonant focus in the same place as the hum.

I use Alexander techniques to get proper alignment, with *Voice and the Alexander Technique* (2005) by Jane Heirich as my primary reference. This fabulous book deals with *habits* and *change*, key elements of re-grooving the SD voice into a functional, typical voice. It also has specific instructions for body alignment to facilitate less restriction to the voice. Movements with sound and visualization techniques are helpful.

Some exercises found in Heirich's book are useful in treating abductor SD because they are designed to "plug up the leaks" using imagery and body movements. Also, using a kazoo or producing the sound "er" gliding up and down scales can be helpful in retraining the vocal folds to be less leaky and the voice to engage more efficiently. Respiratory support without pushing helps minimize these types of spasms as well. Often a person unconsciously pushes through their breathy breaks, which only exacerbates the symptoms.

Ingo Titze, PhD, developed a technique with straws that, "by creating a semi-occluded vocal tract (created by vocalizing through small straws) the static pressure in the mouth and pharynx, spread the vocal folds apart, thereby inviting less collision of the folds" (Titze 2002). For those with AD/SD, it is helpful to vocalize through tiny cocktail straws to allow the adductory muscles of the vocal folds to relax. Dr. Titze suggests doing glides up and down various pitches and then increasing the diameter of the straws. The resistance in this technique also works the respiratory muscles. While described as a warm-up for singers, it can be quite helpful in opening up the throat and pharynx, relaxing the folds, and freeing up the voice in AD/SD patients. Dr. Titze suggests producing the sounds "u," as in shoe, "w," and "y" with and without the straw. A person should go up and down various pitches with the straw, and then remove it, doing the same.

I use Lessac-Madsen Resonant Voice Therapy (LMRVT) techniques as developed by Katherine Verdolini Abbott, PhD, (2008) to help our patients achieve resonance, but I do not use the program materials such as the sessions or home assignments. I use the basic tenants of the program because resonant voice is not a luxury but a necessity, especially in adductor SD. LMRVT aims to decrease the adduction or closure of the vocal folds to "barely touching" to create easy, resonant voice. The use of a lot of nasal consonants, chanting, and humming into words and phrases are all helpful. We discuss the importance of basic vocal hygiene as outlined in the program. This includes issues such as management of gastric reflux, need for hydration, and healthy daily habits in voice use.

I attended Dr. Verdolini's training in 2007 and a master's level class with Professor Arthur Lessac and Dr. Mark Madsen in 2010. Speech therapists are required to attend training before using the LMRVT program. However, many speech pathologists are already trained (listed under practitioners), and a schedule of trainings offered is listed at www.multivoicedimensions.org.

The voice *must* become resonant for SD to be overcome. With symptoms of SD, increased ease in voice production is a challenge. I believe that the faulty sensory signals a person with SD receives are difficult for the body to ignore; hence, many maladaptive habits come into play. Just getting an anchor, such as an easy resonant hum, and returning to it over and over can be an excellent tool for re-grooving. To this day, if my voice begins to feel tight, I just hum a bit and place my voice there as I speak. Another excellent description of vocal resonance can be found in *The Voice Book* by DeVore and Cookman (2009). It is a good overall reference for voice production and exercises for voice improvement with an accompanying CD that is an excellent morning warm-up for any voice.

Very often, yet not always, the pitch of the SD voice is a far cry from a person's optimal pitch range. An optimal pitch range is a person's natural pitch according to the anatomy and physiology of the larynx and free from extraneous tensions and compensations. In my case, my voice went very low in pitch and was quite tremulous. In my attempts to force it to behave, I developed an odd resonance with a low larynx that sounded as if I were talking in a box. Needless to say, I had a lot of tension, poor posture, anxiety, and panic. I could not hum well, sing, or speak. It seemed my voice had deserted me.

The harder I tried, the worse my voice became. Dr. Cooper told me I was speaking too low and that I needed to raise my pitch. During the two days I was with him, I worked primarily on pitch, using *mmm-hmm* and counting to try to correct that. I had discovered that talking to young children and pets was easier for me than speaking to adults and that when I would laugh into a phrase, it would come out more easily and clearly. These were natural anchors to recovering my natural pitch.

I try to establish an optimal pitch for clients very quickly because it is a key element to recovery for the majority of those with SD. I find that if a person can hum easily, it is typically at the optimal pitch. However, if a person hums as if singing or with much tension, the natural pitch will falter. The Cooper Instant Voice Press© may be helpful here; this is quick jabs to the solar plexus while humming. In the case of extreme diaphragm lock, as I call it, the voice press can create a release and allow air to move, relaxing the vocal folds and unleashing the natural pitch. The solar plexus area needs to remain loose and flexible to allow the diaphragm to move and the vocal folds to vibrate freely. To locate it, find the lower ribs with your fingers and walk the fingers upward to the center point. Quick jabs to this area with two fingers or kneading it firmly will loosen it and result in a more natural sound. Tension in this area restricts breath and voice production.

A kazoo is another tool to find optimal pitch. I find that when patients are able to disconnect communicating with the voice, as in humming, the natural pitch is easier to find. A kazoo can do this almost immediately. Of the patients I have treated, including the long-term, severely voice-impaired or those with aphonia, all can produce a normal tone with a kazoo. Then, they can remove the kazoo and reveal the natural pitch with "ooo."

Of course, people don't speak on one pitch. If, for example, a female is speaking at 158 Hz and discovers her optimal pitch to be 220 Hz, we can target that in the hum and with vowels, and then try to keep the practice phrases around that target. We use the Estill Voiceprint ©, Estill Voice International, LLC, program to help people visualize and hear the new target pitch. A computer screen also shows resonance and noise in the voice signal. Mental effort needs to change the habit once the automatic pitch has established itself. Many patients resist this until they hear it enough to realize how much better it sounds than the SD voice. For example, if a person says, "I have an easy time speaking to my dog" I ask that he or she speak that way although the person may resist or feel unusual speaking in that tone. We often explore together the change in the pitch while doing so, with the help of many speaking samples. For information on purchasing this wonderful tool, go to www.EstillVoice.com.

E. *Mindbody Connection*

From the beginning of my voice deterioration, I questioned how my psyche might be influencing my inability to speak. I did not understand what was going on in my body, and I looked in various directions for insight. I truly believe that our bodies have the ability to heal from most diseases. It made sense that my voice disorder could also be healed if I understood and managed it well. I held to the belief that I was simply in a state of dysfunction that could be restored to wellness. This approach to healing is always addressed at our clinics. It encompasses many of the tenants for the psychological and whole body pieces of the SD puzzle and aims to pull them together for more powerful healing potential.

Pre-clinic questionnaires address the time of onset, trauma, stress, and more. Counseling is a large part of the clinic process but may not be the main issue. At times, misuse of the voice is a larger part, and one that typically can be identified easily and quickly. But whether the problem is more psychological or physiological, we are ready to address the issues. We aim to balance the sympathetic (SNS) and the parasympathetic nervous systems (PNS), so that the

PNS is more dominant. The SNS represents our "fight or flight" default and, whether before or after the onset of voice dysfunction, this is the part of the nervous system that quickly becomes in charge. Days with dysfunctional voice become days of repeated panic attacks. When your voice does not work, and you have no idea what will happen when you try to speak, you do **panic**! In a typical day, you panic over and over. When the phone or doorbell ring, when asked a question, when you have to give your phone number, credit card number, food order, directions, and so on...you panic each time you are required to speak. This sets up the "fight or flight reaction." Stress chemicals run wildly through the body until eventually the adrenal glands can become so exhausted, they simply cease to provide the correct balance of chemicals.

What we aim to do at the clinics is to restore the parasympathetic response. The relaxation response is used to relax, release, digest, and heal. It is a state of calmness. Body chemistry changes in this state. The voice relaxes and is easier to produce. As the body relaxes, the heart rate and breath rate decrease. Muscle tension releases. The feel-good chemicals in the body release. People sometimes find that when they first awake from a good sleep or have a few alcoholic beverages, their voice production is more normal. I believe this happens because the nervous system is calmed. A person must learn to trigger this calmness in natural and longer lasting ways through cognitive and behavioral changes and possibly with diet changes or supplements.

Specific breathing reflex triggers allow relaxation to happen quickly and naturally. There are mindbody exercises that increase awareness and allow adjustments by changing the thoughts that are happening moment by moment. We teach positive affirmations and ways to realize that stressors and triggers can take the voice hostage. We teach how to capture those triggers in the moment and change the response so the voice is not taken hostage. We can free the voice if we realize the connection of the trigger and response, and surrender in the moment or return to our anchor.

F. *Group Dynamics*

While individual consultations can be very helpful and are often successful, the group dynamics that the clinics offer are priceless. Because SD is so rare, many people have never met another who understands the emotional ramifications of living with a broken voice. They are especially encouraged by each other along the path. For perhaps the first time, they can relax and speak without the fear of being judged. They also know that my voice was bad for many months, and that I remember intimately the anxiety and fear as well as the questions that ran through my mind from the time of onset to the successful management of my condition. They are free to voice their fears and frustrations to an empathetic group. There are tears and laughter, both easy outlets for the voice. I often tell them they learn as much from each other as they do from me and the team.

G. *Other Voice Development Techniques*

I described several techniques in my original book that may require further explanation. *Voice function exercises, as explained, can be impractical and boring for some because many do not have access to a keyboard to target various pitches. It is difficult to motivate oneself to sustain tones and imagine how this might help them communicate better. We use Roger Love's *Set Your Voice Free* © book and CD as an acceptable substitute for these exercises. Love has a set of exercises on CD that go up and down scales using syllables such as "goog" and "moom." When practiced with an exaggeration of articulation (full excursion of the jaw or fully rounded lips), the end result is an excellent vocal workout similar to the Vocal Function exercises. I do not find sustaining tones to be helpful, but glides from lowest to highest tone are a good workout. Using the Estill Voiceprint program©, a person can track the expansion of range from low to high.

Using exaggerated intonation, or adding a singsong quality to the voice, is helpful. Any tremor is diminished and voice breaks are minimized once a person frees the voice to move around more. It may help to think of your optimum or natural pitch and move up and down from it with more emphasis on the movement than the target. A monotone voice will bring more attention to any voice instability. If the voice gets locked into a limited pitch range, it sounds more strained and stilted. Love has a description of "speak like you sing" in his book and if you sing a phrase then speak it in a similar manner, it can be quite freeing. It also helps to smile and move, using your hands to make gestures as you speak.

Inhalation voicing* can be a helpful technique for a person experiencing many voice breaks or stops. It virtually eliminates these, but to use this manner of voicing in conversation calls negative attention to the speaker and undue stress and feeling of handicap as well. It is meant to be a temporary jump-start to normal vocal fold vibration. In inhalation voicing, speak a word or phrase while inhaling, then immediately say the same on the exhale. Seek to drop the inhalation phonation as soon as possible. It may help to simply *think* of speaking the phrase on an inhale and then speak normally. It serves to break the anticipatory anxiety and the block as well as open up the throat and the channel for the voice. It also prepares for speaking since a person will naturally inhale while preparing to vocalize.

Confidential voice*, or speaking very softly with a bit of a breathy quality, can decrease the effort required in speaking. This is more appropriate for those with adductor SD, but some patients with abductor SD who are using too much effort to try to push the voice out can also find relief with this method. Most abductor patients and some adductor patients have a tendency to give in to whispering very often. This is a big mistake! Whispering does not promote healthy voice production. Whispering is actually not a normal vibratory pattern for the vocal folds but rather a harsh brushing of the folds. In abductor SD, whispering simply reinforces the leaky pattern of voicing and in adductor it may feel easier but will never develop normal vibratory patterns. I recommend not whispering at all.

Any technique that a person finds is an easy outlet for the voice, such as laughing into a phrase or yawning into a phrase is helpful because it is an exploration of the voice. A person can usually find some way to produce an easy and free voice and then use that as their anchor to develop a new groove. Even if the new voice feels fake, it is acceptable. It will not feel that way forever.

*Note that these techniques are not original ideas of the author, and that the specific references are in my initial publication. These techniques were described in earlier publications, and I found them via my personal research on the subject of voice recovery. All are commonly described in various texts on voice therapy.

Chapter 13

Theoretical Model of Neuroplasticity in Successful Voice Rehabilitation

As I worked through my own voice rehabilitation, I would note how my voice would slip in and out of a good groove and how important proper breath support, resonance, and focus were. I had to make adjustments often. The automatic voice I had before was not a good one. Over time, however, I was more in the good groove and less in the bad. I really did move from a voice prison into being free to speak. Still, years later, I find there are days I need to manage my problem. There is an internal struggle around speaking, often not evident to anyone but myself. It may start with a restless night or allergies or even a depressed mood. I may feel as if I don't want to speak. Then what follows might be a day of perceived effort in speaking. If I over-think this issue, I might avoid a conversation or put off a phone call, and the negative spiral can cause more problems. Rarely will this actually have a measurable effect on the acoustics of my voice, but it does require some mental work to maintain control of the voice. I learned that if I record my voice and listen to it, it almost always sounds acceptable. It makes me wonder if the issue of SD is more sensory (felt) than motor and if our reactions to how it feels are what break down voice production so that it gets off groove. Clearly, the more one worries about how he or she sounds, the worse the voice is.

In *The Mind and the Brain: Neuroplasticity and the Power of Mental Force* by Jeffrey Schwartz and Sharon Begley (2002), there is clear evidence of the brain's ability to be rewired throughout life, and how the mind (thoughts) and actions result in significant and lasting changes in the neural pathways. Dr. Schwartz worked with patients with obsessive compulsive disorder (OCD), which had been linked to abnormal activity in certain parts of the brain. Through cognitive-behavioral therapy, these patients got better **and** their brain activity changed. These changes were all documented using fMRI studies.

Brain studies from the National Institutes of Health (NIH) implicated this same issue in people with SD, and the topic was a huge focus of the National Spasmodic Dysphonia Association (NSDA). (Simoyan & Ludlow, 2008) The activity in brains of those with SD symptoms was different from that of normal speakers, and when Botox worked to produce a more fluent voice, the activity again changed. The problem with Botox was that it allowed for changes when it worked, and it was temporary. I thought, "Well, I will use the intention of my mind to make the necessary behavioral and cognitive changes and recover my voice by finding a new groove." And so, in time, I did. But of course, since the brain is always changing, the off groove can also try to work its way back in. I have gone from months to a year or more giving little thought to speaking, then I struggle for days or weeks. The difference now is that I can always produce an acceptable voice, and I don't worry that my voice will get out of control. A decent voice is just a few minor adjustments away.

The *feeling* of effort in voice production is my main problem now, and it is not consistently present. My friends, many who are speech pathologists, perceive my voice to be completely normal and will reinforce that by telling me how nicely resonant my voice sounds. When the specialists come into the picture, they are often looking for problems. SD is considered to be incurable, so it is an issue of debate whether I still have the disorder. If I do still have it, how can my voice sound normal? At the Voice Symposium, Dr. Christy Ludlow said to me, "I hear a lot of adductory breaks in your voice" and I had to reply, "Well, you would." I do not have adductory breaks in my voice. At its worst, I may lack resonance or my voice might be a bit shaky, usually from nervousness. Most people would agree that my voice does not sound unusual. Acoustic analysis indicates normal parameters. Most specialists in SD are not interested in the positive attributes of my voice. To acknowledge that I have a good voice would mean to accept the holistic rehabilitation model as a valid treatment method. When I work with people who have SD, their reactions are the absolute opposite. They think my voice is wonderful because I speak freely without obvious struggle and actually enjoy talking. They can see and hear video and audio samples of my days with SD and, by doing so, see where their efforts can take them. I have recovered. I still have SD. I simply wish that the specialists would accept the positive changes that have occurred in my voice and the improvements in the lives and voices of others.

To achieve rehabilitation does not have to mean a perfect voice. Few humans are blessed with a consistently perfect voice. But recovering from SD means to no longer let the voice handicap you, to manage day to day, to come to self-acceptance, and to find your new groove. It means that your voice does not define who you are and that you can fearlessly speak in all situations. You can ignore or laugh at the little blips you may continue to experience from time to time and literally "go with the flow" that you rediscover with your voice. If a person does not learn to focus on what is right with the voice and accept something shy of "perfect," it is difficult to change.

Some people say they do not want to have to change their voices, and they resist this. Their resistance will hold them back if they attempt voice rehabilitation. Of course, every person with SD wants to recreate that feeling of ease and effortless speaking they remember. It can happen, but it may not always be effortless. There is the choice of having Botox treatment, which requires no work, but will change the voice temporarily. However, if a person is willing to make changes in voice production under his or her own volition, this will result in more permanent changes with or without Botox.

Neuroplasticity theories continue to abound. Norman Doidge, MD, a psychiatrist and researcher, has written a fantastic book on the subject, *The Brain That Changes Itself* (2007), with profound stories of success in the human brain's ability to switch genes on and off and alter our brain anatomy, rewiring many aspects of the brain that control the body. He has award-winning videos, and he lectures frequently on this subject.

If voice rehabilitation is going to work in the long-term for a significant number of those with SD, we must accept the reality that it can be done. SD patients have felt victimized by the very ones meant to treat them for a long time. Well-meaning professionals have told us that our voices are held captive by irregular signals from our brains, and we can do nothing to change the condition other than rely on paralyzing injections to control muscle movement. Recent neuroplasticity evidence presents a very different picture. I wish I had been given this good news at the onset of my diagnosis. It is certainly what I was looking for, and I believe it would have made for an easier transition. It certainly would have spared me some of the trauma and desperation I felt. I was not expecting a fatalistic view of my "incurable" condition and the suggestion of a quick jab of toxin in the neck to relieve my symptoms. I am so thankful that I chose to take my voice under my own control, and that I was blessed to have found a way out.

In essence, recovery from SD means taking personal responsibility for finding one's way out and a knowing deep within one's being that change is possible. Recovery cannot begin if time is wasted without a proper diagnosis or if all treatment options are not honestly discussed. Botox can be a valid treatment option but it is not the cure or the end of SD. Sometimes a medical professional who has not experienced the devastation of voice loss will downplay the emotional agony of the disorder and simply prescribe Botox injections as the gold standard of treatment it has become. It would be in the patients' best interest to understand what Botox can and cannot do and combine with that the possibility that other avenues are available, either with or without drug treatment.

If a person truly wants to beat SD, it has to come from within, using the tools one is given or finds. The tools must include a daily routine of strategies to change the faulty patterns that have become automatic in the brain. Of course, relieving symptoms with Botox injections is a personal choice, and it is not my intention to discredit or disprove it. For some, it may be better to give their control over to a medical model, or it might be necessary. I do not have all the answers, but I do have my experience and the experiences of those I treat as firm evidence that an alternative exists. All the years of "failures" of voice therapy are simply because we did not know how to treat the disorder.

I just received an email from a client who came to us from Finland. She is not included in the case studies in the book. Her recovery was a **real** adventure, so I'd like to close with her email message. It came at the perfect time. "Masi" was diagnosed in September 2008 with adductor SD after a two-year slow deterioration of her voice. She attended the clinic in January 2009. Her VHI score was 93. Her symptoms were also severe, but she improved significantly at the clinic. Unfortunately, she had a recurrence of breast cancer, and her voice declined during the process of fighting the disease. Two months ago, she informed me that she was 90 percent recovered with her voice and had also recovered from her metastatic breast cancer. She felt that the strategies she learned here, changing occupations, chiropractic adjustments, and recovery of her self-esteem allowed her recovery. On June 13, 2010, she emailed, "Thank you for your newsletter. You gave me faith, and now I am running my own company (nutrition and life blood analysis). Whatever the degenerative disease a person has is a mind body spirit connection. A person is what he thinks, breathes, eats, and drinks. I now speak 2 hours per customer, sometimes 5 customers a day. I am planning lectures at the university in the fall. I have customer events and use my voice extensively. All this after SD and metastatic breast cancer, which I think are in the PAST. Thank you for practicing (Mahatma Ghandi's quote) **'Be the change you wish to see in the world.'** You have done this and I want to do the same."

I'm thankful that Masi's email came to me on a Sunday afternoon as I pondered how to end this chapter with a poignant message. The big message for those with SD is **hope**! It is real, recovery is real, and neuroplasticity is the reason. For professionals treating those with SD, do **not** take away hope and do **not** practice negativity lest the nocebo effect take over your patient's mindbody. Please be honest about the limitations of any treatment that does not address the mind's intention and personal responsibility for change. For people suffering with SD, there is hope for healing and re-grooving your voice. Please know that you, too, can be free to speak again. There is no time limit; just let go of limiting and gripping minds, and gain strategies from open and innovative professionals who will believe in you! I believe in you and in the message this book brings.

Chapter 14

The Future of Holistic Intensive Rehabilitation of SD

Earlier this summer (2010), I decided to tiptoe into the scientific voice professional world. I attended the Voice Symposium and was perceived as pesky as a fly at a picnic. I had been working on an NIH grant the previous month, putting my book project and clinics on hold. The proposal was exciting. The National Institutes of Health along with the National Institute on Deafness and Communication Disorders was offering a grant opportunity for innovative methods and promising therapeutic approaches to treat spasmodic dysphonia. It seemed tailored to my program and so, with great excitement, I downloaded all the necessary application materials and set sail. I hoped to be able to attain grant money to fund the clinic fees for SD patients over an eighteen to twenty-four month period so that I could apply a more rigorous scientific study to establish efficacy. This might lead to further grants to provide training to other speech pathologists. I began the arduous process, seeking guidance along the way from those more savvy with government grants.

I became increasingly discouraged when I could find no one "qualified" to collaborate on the project. I lacked the qualifications and experience to be considered a researcher. I was not affiliated with a university or hospital and I did not have the educational qualifications, specifically a PhD. It quickly became clear to me that I was out of my league. Without an established collaborator, my grant application would have no chance of consideration. How silly of me to think I had the credentials to join such a league of research scientists. Seasoned researchers and those serving on the very committees that read these grants advised me not to submit the grant application at this time.

I began to explore what **really** mattered to me. Was it to be accepted by the scientific community? From what I observed at the Voice Symposium, I decided I did not care to be accepted if it compromised my own recovery because of the added stress or interfered in my work helping people with SD. I didn't need to prove myself or my methods because they have been clearly established with efficacy data and case studies. My methods are not a farce or quick fix or "cure" for spasmodic dysphonia. But they are proving to be successful management tools for improving this condition, especially rendering many people less handicapped as a result. Some have regained normal voice production. With great heaviness of heart, I abandoned the grant project. I still have all the materials in a bright blue three-inch binder to remind me of my effort. The project is online and partially ready for submission, but this is not the right time. This book took precedence and I began to schedule clinics again.

A few professionals are interested in coauthoring or collaborating on a future journal article with a theoretical focus. Perhaps the publication of this book will spark more interest. Professionals might better accept a slower introduction to my theory and treatment, and consider a journal article a more realistic goal than a grant proposal. I have to remember all the pioneers from history that were shunned, jailed, or even killed for trying to change an established paradigm and be thankful that skepticism, criticism, and lack of grant support are probably the worst outcomes for me.

I know that my consciousness of and my care for those who suffer with SD must be the main focus. I feel compelled to continue to treat those with SD using this holistic program because I know it works. I will continue to offer the clinics and publicly outline the key aspects of voice rehabilitation for individuals suffering from spasmodic dysphonia as well as to professionals treating it. If a people can afford only this book, with no funding for private consultation or a clinic, I hope that the ending chapter will help guide them on their way to finding a way out of this debilitating illness and move toward speaking freely once again.

Chapter 15
Suggested Program of Intensive Holistic Voice Rehabilitation for SD

Engaging in a program of voice rehabilitation should only be done after obtaining medical clearance and it is best accomplished with the guidance of a certified speech pathologist. It is difficult to acquire the right exercises and do them correctly on your own. These suggested exercises are not meant to take the place of adequate medical care and therapy. SD is a very individual disorder and different for virtually every person who suffers from it. If a person takes on the suggested exercises in the light of self-exploration, using what helps and letting go of what does not, the process can result in big changes and improvements in voice production. It is possible that in addition to these suggestions, a mental health professional, massage therapist, yoga instructor, Alexander teacher, chiropractor, nutritionist, naturopath, acupuncturist, or other professional can be highly beneficial. It is important to view recovery as a healing journey that is your own.

Intensive Holistic Voice Rehabilitation has the goal of "doing no harm" and incorporating the mind, body, and spirit into a self-discovery of a new way of living, which leads to a new way of speaking.

A. **Mental and Physical Preparation**

When you decide to embark on a cognitive-behavioral program such as this, it is important to engage fully in the process and not give over personal power to anyone else to provide the "cure." The changes that occur are internal changes, and those changes will become more fully grooved in over time. When desperate, it is easy to fall prey to claims that someone or something will fix you. Even the gold standard of treatment, Botox, will never cure you. It can certainly help with your symptoms, sometimes dramatically. So if Botox is your choice of treatment, choose it with your full intention of what it can and cannot do. You may be able to function well with this treatment, and you may lack the time and self-responsibility for voice rehabilitation. It is still a valid choice.

When you choose voice rehabilitation, understand that it may not be a quick fix. If your SD is inappropriately diagnosed and what you are experiencing is a psychosomatic manifestation or functional dysphonia, very rapid and complete recovery can be expected. It is better to prepare yourself for true SD, however, which will require time and effort in a holistic program to change. In neurological SD, a perfect voice may not be the result of even the best efforts. Improvement is possible in virtually all cases, significant improvement in more than 85 percent. You have a good chance of attaining a voice that is less handicapping and more functional if you comply with the program.

Accept that the mind has the ability to change the brain and that voice production must be understood and embraced. Many books in the reference section provide scientific proof of this phenomenon. Do not believe you are incurable; let go of that idea completely. It is quite possible to re-groove your voice so that it feels easier and sounds better. SD is a manageable condition for most people.

A healthy body will serve you better with regard to overall change and the stamina to do what it takes. Examine your lifestyle and state of health. Do you have many health challenges? Are you significantly overweight, chronically fatigued, or clinically depressed? Are you giving your body plenty of nutritional healthy foods, and are you hydrating well? Are you engaging in physical exercise regularly but not obsessively or in an overly strenuous program? Are you prepared to address these issues prior to engaging in voice rehabilitation? In preparation for voice rehabilitation, it would be in your best interest to have a physical examination. To attend a clinic, you must have medical clearance that includes examination of your vocal folds to rule out any pathological causes for your voice problems. If you have any chronic medical problems, you should seek to manage them in accordance with your physician's suggestions.

Mental health is also very important. A psychosocial profile is included in our clinic and is the first introduction to mental health for many of our clients. A high percentage of our clients are significantly depressed or anxious or both. Some may require counseling or medication to control these issues. Some of our "failures" were clearly those whose mental state would not allow them to take control of making changes, including voice changes. Examine your history for times when you were "not able to express yourself" or current feelings of "not having a voice or being heard." If you lack self-discipline and do not believe you are capable of making positive changes in your life as a whole, it may be difficult for you to engage in voice rehabilitation. Issues of stress have a huge impact on the voice. Are you aware of being "stressed out" and, if so, are you willing to make positive changes to reduce your stress? Is your job toxic, and are you willing to change jobs to find one that suits your personality better? Does your job require high voice use, and do you resent or dread that? Can you take a job leave to complete a program of voice rehabilitation? Some people have been granted short-term disability, which has allowed them to make the necessary cognitive-behavioral changes to free the voice. I took a self-funded leave of absence for eight months to do this. It was priceless in the end, although it required a few sacrifices in the interim. If you think you may be suffering from depression, I would suggest reading *Unstuck* (Gordon 2008). It contains a questionnaire that targets depressed thinking patterns and is a fabulous resource for dealing with depression with a myriad of strategies.

Try engaging in activities that help to develop a calm state. These include gentle exercise, such as walking, swimming, or biking, yoga, Tai Chi, Qigong, meditation, prayer, watching or reading comedy, serving others while maintaining time for oneself, journaling, adequate sleep, healthy foods, and nutritional supplements. Daily relaxation time is important. Sleep and watching TV are not a substitute because neither consciously quiet the mind nor relax the muscles.

Just a few notes on nutrition: Overall, strive for a healthy diet that nurtures your body. Avoid Aspartame®; it is a proven neurotoxin and is found in Diet colas. (Brackett and Waldron 2004). Watch your acidity level—you need to eat more alkaline foods like fresh fruits and vegetables. Generally, minimize processed foods and additives such as MSG. Regular elimination (bowel movements) is crucial for overall health. This can be easily managed with diet and natural supplements. Stay hydrated and ingest plenty of water all day and into the evening hours. For more information, ask your doctor for a diet plan or visit a nutritional expert.

Understand the medications you are being prescribed as well as the side effects they may have on your voice. Many pharmaceutical drugs can prolong your life, improve your quality of life, and possibly even save it. However, a pill is not the answer for every health issue you face. Be your own advocate and explore holistic medicine. Know your drugs. Physical and mental preparation may seem like a strange place to start working on the voice, but it is necessary and should be the **first** place to start.

B.   **Breathing Development**

For the first five years of the clinic, Mike White used his Optimal Breathing program, providing the breathing coaching as well as nutritional counseling. His website contains a plethora of information on breathing development, and he offers various programs, breathing enhancement devices, and nutritional supplements. At the time of publication, Dennis Price, a prior student of Mike's and also a skilled life coach, neuromuscular therapist, and Certified Neurolinguistic Programming Specialist, is serving in this role.

In most cases of SD, breathing patterns are very poor. It is not clear whether or not SD is a result of poor breathing or a consequence, but the more people I treat, the more I feel that it is the latter. My reasoning is that I observe many people breathing poorly who produce good speaking voices. However, based on my own experience, at the onset of SD, breathing dynamics usually deteriorate. Perhaps this is stress-induced. Stress activates the sympathetic nervous system, resulting in rapid, shallow breathing. SD is a major stressor, often preceded by multiple stressors. Perhaps it is due to the sensation of difficulty with voice production, for which we compensate by attempts to push the voice out using our stomach muscles. We gasp and heave and are very inefficient with coordinating the breath with the voice. Rarely do I see someone with SD who has a good breathing pattern, at least with regard to speaking.

It is clear that developing good breathing techniques is a crucial part of the program. I have researched the literature on breathing development, and much of what I have read is simply not good practice for producing a voice with minimal effort. Diaphragmatic breathing is often prescribed and trained, but the way it is done can be contraindicated once the breath and voice need to be coordinated. For example, the following exercises are excellent for developing diaphragmatic or abdominal breathing and will progress from quiet breathing to breathing for speech:

1. Lying down on a firm surface, place one hand on your stomach and one on your chest. As you inhale, or take in a breath, you should feel only your stomach move. It should move outward against your hand. As you exhale, you should feel the stomach move inward, finally pulling

it inward to exhale all the breath. The last sentence applies to developing breathing technique but **not** to speaking.

2. In a seated or supported position, repeat the above. Inhale, stomach moves out; exhale, stomach moves inward. Pause and repeat.

3. A possibly better exercise is the Squeeze and Breathe exercise described in my first book and on Mike's website. Standing, with thumbs to the back and fingers wrapped around the sides at the level of the navel, squeeze the hands together. Take a big inhalation with the intention of pushing the fingers away from the thumb, opening your grasp with the breath. Take as big a breath in as you can, focusing on moving your hands apart, and keeping the shoulders level. It is important not to move the shoulders or chest as you do this. Release the breath and try again. If this is difficult, do it repeatedly throughout every day until it begins to feel more coordinated and the movement in the abdomen becomes bigger.

4. The main change in breathing for voice production is what happens on the exhalation. The "push" of the stomach muscles to force the air out is contraindicated when speaking. A passive exhalation is all that is needed to vibrate the vocal folds. If the air is pushed out with tension in the stomach, two things can happen. In adductor SD, any push from the stomach causes the vocal folds to press more tightly together such as in the Valsalva maneuver previously described. Voice breaks and stops can occur. Voice production becomes more like a grunt and sounds strangled. In abductor SD, the push from the stomach muscles blows the vocal folds open so that a rush of air precedes voicing or prolongs voiceless consonants. There is a

distinct connection between the activity of the abdominals in exhalation and in the behavior of the vocal folds in SD. For those who do not have SD symptoms, the abdominal activity does not play such a role, and singers often use these muscles effectively.

5.   Humming is often the easiest way to establish normal vocal fold production from a breathing perspective. Breathe in but not to the fullest extent that you can, as too much air in the lungs is contraindicated. Keeping the stomach **out**, and stomach muscles loose, hum. Place a hand on the stomach to be sure that it stays soft. If you continue to feel the stomach muscles tighten as you hum, then a *slight* push out toward your hand can counteract that.

6.   Humming is a good starting place for coordinating the breath with the voice. If you cannot easily hum, using a kazoo can be helpful. Remember that it requires an engagement of the voice to make an "oooo" rather than simply blowing air. Go for easy sound, soft stomach. If you are having difficulty humming, read on.

C.   **Unraveling Muscular Tension and Establishing Proper Posture**

The purpose of this section is not to make an argument or attempt differential diagnosis of muscle tension dysphonia (MTD) and spasmodic dysphonia. I believe that too much time and energy is devoted to providing the correct diagnosis, and I have seen a shift from the time not long ago when a person diagnosed with MTD would be treated only with voice therapy and possibly laryngeal massage. Currently, those with MTD are often referred for Botox treatment to release the tension. Many patients with SD develop terrible compensations for the disorder, which involve muscle tension. This is a crucial area of exploration. Some speech therapists are skilled at identifying and treating laryngeal muscle tension. Not all people with SD have extremely tight laryngeal muscles but many do. Our neuromuscular therapist is very skilled at identifying and treating muscle imbalances and tension in the face, tongue, throat, chest, thoracic area, rib cage, and diaphragm.

1. Seek out a neuromuscular therapist or a speech therapist trained in laryngeal massage. Manipulation of the position of the larynx in the neck can be very helpful and immediately free up the voice to some degree. Techniques for laryngeal massage are described by Roy et al. (1997) and, more recently, Mathieson et al. (2009).
2. Examine the tension in your face and neck daily. Examine yourself breathing and speaking in a mirror. Do you see a furrowed brow, a frown, tight lips, raised shoulders? Is your head jutted forward or held back or down as a turtle going into its shell? Look at your posture from a side angle. Is your head stable and positioned so that your neck and chin appear as an upside down "L" or is your angle too open or closed? Never practice or speak while looking down. Maintain an upside down "L" as you speak, especially on the phone.
3. Try these simple exercises to loosen up the face and lips: trill the lips in a "brrrr," trill the tongue in a "trrrr." Don't worry if you can't do both, or either. Simply **relax** the lips and tongue as much as possible and do it without voicing if that is easier. Use sloppy talk, "blah, blah, blah," opening your mouth as widely as comfortable on the "ah" and

sticking your tongue out for the "la." Massage your cheeks with the palms of your hands.

4. Do neck stretches daily. Tilt the head slightly to the right, pulling gently with the right hand on the top of your head. Repeat to the left. Drop the chin to the chest and roll the chin right to left in semicircles.

5. Attend to the musculature under your chin. If you hum or speak and you feel a bulging of the muscles under your chin, it may be inhibiting the resonance of your voice. Work to free up this muscle by massaging it and humming with the intention of keeping it relaxed. It is attached to the tongue so those exercises are also helpful.

6. Attend to your body posture. Is your spine straight? (Yoga is wonderful for body alignment and highly recommended). Try standing against a wall, then stepping away, still in alignment. Think "down to go up." This is an Alexander lesson. Commit your feet to the earth or your bottom to your seat, feet engaged with the earth. Allow the full length of your spine to move upward as if a string were attached to the top of your head, pulling it toward the ceiling.

7. For best voice production, shoulders should not round. Chest should be open and not collapse. Spread your arms **wide**. Wrap them around your back and try to grab opposite elbows, feeling the openness in the front of your body. Hum now; is it easier?

8. Pay close attention to your diaphragm. I find it is often "frozen" or stiff in those with SD and impedes proper breath flow. Place your hands flat, right on top of left, under the **center** of your rib cage and pull your elbows close to your body. Inhale deeply, pushing your body toward your hands

and hands back toward your body. Hold your breath and push hard. Release, relax, and repeat three times. Then on an in-breath, reach your right hand around the left side of your waist, fingers spread; on the out-breath, pull your fingers to your navel with pressure. Repeat two times and then work with the left hand/right side. You've just freed the diaphragm in about a minute (Eden, 1998). It can also help to poke, knead, or make circular movements in this area.

D. Voice Exercises

1. Once an easy, effortless hum is established, it can become the bridge to easier voicing. The aim is to have a vibration along the roof of the mouth and out the front of the face while vocalizing. With AD/SD, I recommend going into resonant voice techniques at this point. Recall the discussion around LMRVT in Chapter 12. The aim is to use the hum to establish optimal pitch range, and then to move into chanting (memememe, mymymymy, momomomo) and then speaking words, phrases, and sentences.

2. Saying a genuine mmm-hmm as if agreeing with someone is a good way to establish pitch. Use of a visualization of pitch can be helpful. I recommend the Estill Voiceprint® program. The pitch produced on a hum or with a kazoo is easily visualized. If you establish this pitch and realize that your speaking voice is much higher or lower, you will need to make some mental adjustments and practice speaking at a different pitch. It is important not to resist this because it feels odd or unnatural. Remember that automatic (what you think is natural) is not working. Voiceprint also allows you to record and play back thirty-second clips for

immediate auditory feedback. Your own ear may not be the best judge of voice acoustics. A recording is best.

3. For those with AB/SD, especially if severely breathy, a resonant hum may be difficult as the air tends to rush out the nose. Saying "er," held out for several seconds, engages the vocal folds better. A kazoo is very helpful. Visualize the vocal folds closing and engaging. Say "ring" and hold out the "ng." This is an open-mouth hum and helps to engage the vocal folds. If there is air escaping through the nose while humming, the open-mouth version inhibits it.

4. Use a yawn to facilitate the voice, especially in AD/SD. Begin with yawn, "ah," and progress to yawning and speaking single words. Later, just imagining a yawn opens up the throat and facilitates voicing.

5. Repetitive right voice use grooves it in. I have developed many word lists with most consonants and vowels. These are prescribed as progressing from easy to hard and are different for AD (typically beginning with m,n,h) than for AB (typically r, long a, ng). You must practice isolated sounds first, and then progress to words, phrases, and sentences as you attain success at each level. This aspect of motor learning is quite important, and you must not move too quickly to the next level or it will result in negative practice. The more you speak in the SD voice, the more it gets grooved in, so this must be avoided. (For some people, a quick shift to normal voice does not require this type of re-grooving. If you can shift into a good voice and use it conversationally, count yourself lucky and keep talking!)

6. Facilitate freedom of voice through singing exercises (such as Roger Love's CD) or hum-speaking technique. Sing or

hum a phrase, then speak it immediately, trying to match the intonation pattern, pitch, and resonance.

7. Use movement to facilitate sound. Breaststroke around the room, speaking as you go. I like to begin with "I talk like this" as a first phrase. Reach one and then the other arm up as if stretching as you speak. Squat down on one knee and rock forward and backward with arms held high as you speak. Hold the arms out in a "T" position and move your whole body right to left so that your arms "slap" your back as you speak a phrase with the movement. The arms must be very loose. Simply, use your hands as you speak. Loosen up!

8. Use exaggerated articulation and intonation. Singsong, with emphasis on various words.
    *Weeeellll, I **wanted** to do it **MYYYYY WAAAY**. Am IIIIII doing it **RIIIIGHT?*** Use very big movements of lips and tongue. Open the mouth **wide** for all the vowels. Try chewing your words as you speak.

9. Attend to where your voice is focused. Most people with AD/SD have the voice focused in the throat, which is a big mistake. It simply increases tension there and does not allow proper vocal fold vibration. Move it upward to the face. Imagery is helpful here. Think of the throat as a musky old basement full of spiders to be avoided. Go upstairs with your voice to the loft, where it is airy and light and full of sunshine and bright colors. Stay in the loft, or at least in the house, but definitely avoid the basement. It is not safe!

10. In the case of AB/SD, the focus is not typically the throat, but the nose. Often air is rushing through the nose as a person attempts to speak. The focus here needs to move

back down to the throat to engage the vocal folds. "Errrr" is an excellent anchor for engaging the vocal folds. Remember to engage without push!

11. Play and experiment with the voice. Many people with SD find that playing around with a different accent or a soft, confidential voice or loud announcer-type voice frees them up. Use this "fake" voice as an *anchor* to convince your mindbody that you really can have a non-SD voice and use it to develop your new groove. Anything goes, as long as it is fun and **easy**.

During rehabilitation, self-care is very important. Minimize talking in SD voice, even if it means delegating voice responsibilities for a time. I find that most people with SD are very talkative, despite their faulty voices. It may be difficult, but you must develop the awareness to inhibit the SD voice and facilitate the freer, clear, and easier voice for the new groove to become established. The need to talk can become almost impulsive and obsessive. Learn to be a quiet listener and to weigh your words carefully during the re-grooving process. Right, repetitive, easy voicing is your way out of SD.

E. **Energy Medicine**

Holistic medicine recognizes energy fields within the human body. These have been a part of Indian and Chinese medicine for many years but only recently embraced in our Western health care system by some professionals. I have recently chosen a holistic medical doctor, Dr. Carol Roberts, to partner in my health care, and it was long overdue. Her book *Good Medicine: A Return to Common Sense* (2010) is a wonderful introduction to the aspects of holistic medicine and contains a chapter on the anatomy of the energy body. In it, she describes the chakra system based on the flow of energy from the ground toward the heavens, which contains seven centers.

While we do not actively practice energy medicine as such in the clinics, we know enough about the chakras and energy fields and meridians to make some contribution. Many body workers, acupuncturists, and holistic physicians are knowledgeable and can help in these areas. For the purpose of voice, the fifth chakra, located in the throat with its center at the hyoid bone and encircling the larynx, is the most important. In Dr. Robert's words, it "concerns itself with self-expression...where one finds her voice, her will, her mission in life. Deficient fifth chakra energy results in feelings of lack, frustration, of the damming up of the natural flow of heart energy upward toward God."

According to Donna Eden, author of *Energy Medicine* (1998), "The two basic behavioral difficulties people have that are connected to the throat chakra are that they can't speak up or they can't shut up." Most people, including myself, can attest to being very talkative until SD reared its ugly head. Interestingly, most people with SD still long to talk and the clinics can be very lively. SD seems to be more common in people who use their voices excessively in their chosen occupations.

The other very important chakra to attend to when you have SD is the third chakra located at the solar plexus. According to Dr. Roberts, "Its theme is acquisition of power. Too much energy can result in arrogance and domination, too little energy here in low self-esteem and lack of confidence." I find that this area can get very tight and sore in most people with SD. They seem to try to push the voice out from here. It is also where the diaphragm is located.

F. Spiritual Aspects of Voice Rehabilitation

I am generally a non-confrontational person, and I joke about staying away from religion or politics as topics of discussion. Spiritual, however, is not the same as religious. I believe we are all spiritual beings; we came of spirit, the Spirit of God breathed life into us, and when we depart our earthly bodies, we once again become spirit.

For me, SD was a spiritual awakening. I happen to be a Christian, but I am much more spiritual than religious. I have friends and patients of virtually all religions or of none, and still there is the spirit that connects us as human beings. I believe that all challenges we encounter in our earth life give us the opportunity to grow. As I was virtually speechless for a time, I became more introspective and had many dialogues with God on the issue of "why me, why this, why now?" Once I regained a healthy voice, it seemed so clear why it had to happen. Of course, I was to teach others, to maybe shift a world paradigm. Then I came to call it a gift.

I still struggle with the spiritual issue of my son's death. I can claim the truth of the Bible and cling to Ecclesiastes 3, "To everything there is a season, and a time to every purpose under heaven. A time to be born, and a time to die." I accept that it was Taylor's time to die. That is hard, but I also know that we all die, these earthly bodies of ours. And I know Taylor's spirit is very much present. We must do our best while we are on earth to make a difference and make the world a better place by our presence. I believe that spirit and love never die, and our contribution to the world matters. That is what we leave when our bodies become dust.

I encourage everyone with SD to consider it a life lesson of sorts. Examine where you are on your spiritual path and how this might work some good in your life. Journal, pray, embrace this time to be introspective. Draw power from your Creator to give you strength and accept healing in every form it takes. In the clinics, we address spirituality to whatever extent it is needed by each person. I am happy to pray with or for anyone. Despite the various religious or spiritual beliefs represented in the group, we are all bound by a common spirit, and it accelerates the healing. It is okay to ask, "why me, why this, why now?" but with the reverence of not being in complete control. There is a sovereignty of the situation, of our Higher Power being in ultimate control, while absolutely wanting the best for us. There is strength to be found here, in spirit. To ignore it would be to set aside a very large part of what makes us who we are.

G. Support

Having a voice problem as severe as SD is extremely isolating. Due to the social and emotional impact this disorder has, it is often very liberating for patients to meet me and realize that successful management is possible and to work through the healing process with others who truly understand how it feels to live life with a broken voice. The clinics provide this support and commonly, people attending a clinic together form close bonds and stay in touch long after the clinic ends. I highly recommend some sort of support resource for all who have SD. If a clinic is not a possibility, local groups are typically created by the NSDA and can be found on their website. A good online resource for all voice disorders is VoiceMatters.org, a wealth of support and information in a non-biased open forum.

In closing, it is not my intention to create an illusion that managing and overcoming SD is an easy task. Your brain is not cooperating with the signals it sends and receives to and from your vocal fold muscles. Various compensations lock up the body or the mind or both. It is a very complex process and can be quite fragile. The emotional consequence of a broken voice is profound. But the good news here is that this faulty pathway can become smooth again, and it can be managed. Believe it and do it. Your body mind will thank you as you become free to speak once again. Whether you jump-start your program with an intensive clinic or you work this program with your own speech pathologist (or your own patients!), I am with you in spirit and look forward to a time when SD has a more positive prognosis and a multitude of successful people who are managing and overcoming it. God Bless You, Namaste, Love, and Light!

References

Ali SO, *et al.* (2006) Alterations in CNS activity induced by botulinum toxin treatment in spasmodic dysphonia: an H2 15 O Pet study. *J Speech Hear Res*; 49: 1127-1146.

Abitbol, J. (2006) *Odyssey of the Voice.* San Diego, Plural Publishing.

American Speech and Hearing Association website (1997-2010). Retrieved from http://www.asha.org/public/speechdisorders/Spasmodic -Dysphonia.htm

Behrad, *et al.* (2010) A single center retrospective review of unilateral and bilateral Dysport® injections in adductor spasmodic dysphonia. *Logo Phonia Voc;* 35; 39-44.

Blitzer, A., *et al.* (1998) Botulinum toxin management of spasmodic dysphonia: a 12 year experience in more than 900 patients. *Laryngoscope;* 108: 1435-1441.

Blitzer, A. (2010) Spasmodic dysphonia and botulinum toxin: experience from the largest treatment series. *Europ J Neur:* 17 (supp 1): 28-30.

Boutsen, F., *et al.* (2002) Botox treatment in Adductor Spasmodic Dysphonia: A Meta-Analysis. *Jour Speech Hear Res;* 45: 469-481.

Brackett, C. & Waldron, J.T. (2004) *Sweet Misery: A poisoned world.* Sound and Fury Productions, Inc.

Braden, *et al* (2008) Assessing the Effectiveness of Botulinum Toxin Injections for Adductor Spasmodic Dysphonia: Clinician and Patient Perception. *Journal of Voice;* 24: 242-249.

Chhetri, D., *et al* (2006) Long-Term Follow-up Results of Selective Laryngeal Adductor Denervation-Reinnervation Surgery for Adductor Spasmodic Dysphonia. *Laryngoscope;* 116: 635-642.

Coelho, P. (2003) *Warrior of the Light: A Manual.* New York, HarperCollins.

Cooper, M. (2006) Curing Hopeless Voices: The Strangled Voice (Spasmodic Dysphonia) & Other Voice Problems with Direct Voice Rehabilitation. © by Morton Cooper, Ph.D. All rights reserved.

DeVore, K. & Cookman, S. (2009) *The Voice Book: Caring for, protecting, and improving your voice.* Chicago, Chicago Review Press.

Doidge, N. (2007) *The Brain that Changes Itself.* New York, Viking, Penguin Group.

Eden, D. (1998) *Energy Medicine.* © by Donna Eden. New York, Most Tarcher/Putnam.

Estill Voiceprint. Estill Voice International, LLC. www.EstillVoice.com.

Epstein, R. (2005) Interview by Stephanie Martin. Retrieved March 1, 2006. http://www.british-voice-association.com/archive/profiles/ruth_epstein.htm.

Federal Drug Administration website. www.fda.gov/Drugs/

Gordon, J. (2008) *Unstuck: Your guide to the seven stage journey out of depression.* New York, The Penguin Press.

Haselden, K. *et al* (2009) Comparing Health Locus of Control in Patients with Spasmodic Dysphonia, Functional Dysphonia and Nonlaryngeal Dystonia. *Journal of Voice*; **23** (6): 699-706.

Heirich, J. (2005) *Voice and the Alexander Technique.* Berkeley, Mortum Time Press.

HY Li, *et al* (2009) Self assessment characteristics of voice handicap index for voice disorders and its influencing factors. MEDLINE abstact http://highwire.stanford.edu/cgi/medline/pmid; 19558882, retrieved 7/03/2009.

Jeffers, S. (1987, 2007) *Feel the Fear and Do It Anyway*, London, Vermilion.

Kasden, M., *et al* (1999) "The Nocebo Effect: Do No Harm", *Jour South Ortho Assoc.*

Langefield, T, *et al* (2001) Evaluation of Voice Quality in adductor spasmodic dysphonia before and after Botox treatment. *Ann Otol Rhinol Larngol;* **110**: 627-634.

Linklater, K. (2006) *Freeing the Natural Voice.* Hollywood, Drama Publishers.

Love, R. (1999) *Set Your Voice Free.* Boston, Little, Brown & Company.

Ludlow, C. (2006) Central Nervous System control of the laryngeal muscles. Author manuscript retrieved June 18, 2006. http://www.pubmedcentral.gov/articles.fcgi?tool=pubmed&pubmedid=15927543

Mathieson, L., *et al* (2009) Laryngeal Manual Therapy: A preliminary study to examine its treatment effects in the management of muscle tension dysphonia. *Journ of Voice*; **23**(3): 353-366.

Munro M., *et al* (2009) Collective Writings on the Lessac Voice and Body Work: A Festschrift, Coral Springs, Lumina Press.

Murray, T., *et al* (1994) Combined-modality treatment of adductor spasmodic dysphonia with botulinum toxin and voice therapy. *Journal of Voice*; **9** (4): 460-465.

National Spasmodic Dysphonia Association website (2000) www. dysphonia.org.

NIH publication, Spasmodic Dysphonia. Retrieved June 26, 2010 http://www.nidcd.nih.gov/health/voice/spasdysp.html.

Parry, W. (2000, 2006) Understanding and Controlling Stuttering: A comprehensive new approach based on the Valsalva hypothesis. © by William Parry, distributed in cooperation with the National Stuttering Association, NY.

Pert, C. (2006) *Everything you need to know to feel Go(o)d*. USA, Hay House, Inc.

Pert, C. *et al* (2004) *Psychosomatic Wellness—Healing your Bodymind* CD package. Magic Bullet Productions.

Pike, C. (2005) *Free to Speak: Overcoming Spasmodic Dysphonia*. Charleston, Booksurge Publishing.

Psychological Publications, Inc. (2007) *Taylor-Johnson Temperament Analysis®*, Thousand Oaks, California.

Reid, B. (2002) "The Nocebo Effect: Placebo's Evil Twin", *The Washington Post,* April 30, 2002.

Roberts, C. (2010) *Good Medicine: A Return to Common Sense*© Carol L. Roberts, M.D., Mercurine Press.

Root-Bernstein, R. (1998) *Honey, Mud Maggots and other Medical Marvels: The Science Behind Folk Remedies and Old Wives' Tales.* Houghton Mifflin.

Roy, N. *et al* (1997) Manual circumlaryngeal therapy for functional dysphonia: An evaluation of short- and long-term treatment outcomes. *Jour of Voice*; 11: 321-331.

Sarno, J. (1991) *Healing Back Pain*, New York, Warner Books.

Sarno, J. (2006) *The Divided Mind: the epidemic of mindbody disorders.* New York, HarperCollins Publishers, Inc.

Schwartz, J. & Begley, S. (2002) *The Mind and the Brain: Neuroplasticity and the Power of Mental Force.* New York, HarperCollins Publishers, Inc.

Stemple, J. (2000) *Voice Therapy: clinical studies.* Clifton Park, NY, Delmar Learning.

Simonyan, K., *et al* (2008) Focal white matter changes in spasmodic dysphonia: a combined diffusion tensor imaging and neuropathological study. *Brain:* 131 (2); 447-459.

Simonyan, K. & Ludlow, C. (2010) Abnormal Activation of the Primary Somatosensory Cortex in Spasmodic Dysphonia: An fMRI study. *Cerebral Cortex.* Advanced Access published online on March 1, 2010. Oxford University Press. Retrieved March 2,

2010. http://cercor.oxfordjournals.org/cgi/content/abstract/bhq02 3v1?maxtoshow=&hits=1&RESULTFORMAT

Titze, I. (2002) How to use flow resistant straws. *Journ of Singing*; **58** (5); 429-430.

Verdolini-Abbott, K. (2008) *Lessac-Madsen Resonant Voice Therapy*, © by Plural Publishing, Inc., San Diego.

Voelker, R. (1996) Nocebos Contribute to a Host of Ills. *Journ Am Med Assoc;* **275** (5); 345-347.

Zeuner, KE, *et al* (2008) Motor re-training does not need to be task specific to improve writer's cramp. *Mov Disord;* DOI 10.1002/ mds.222222. Published online September 24, 2008. Retrieved December 30, 2008.

Vidailhet, M., *et al* (2004) The benefit of MEG and fMRI and neurophysiology in understanding dystonia. *Rev neurol* (Paris): **160** (1), 1S13-1S14.

Voice Matters website (2008) www.voicematters.net